Sixty
is a
Good
Start

A Powerful Body, a Purposeful Life,
and a Plan to Make It Happen

Sixty
is a
Good
Start

A Powerful Body, a Purposeful Life,
and a Plan to Make It Happen

Allison McCune Davis

Niche Pressworks
Indianapolis, IN

Sixty Is a Good Start
Copyright © 2025 by Allison McCune Davis

This book is written as a source of information only. The information contained in this book should by no means be considered a substitute for the advice of a qualified medical professional, who should always be consulted before beginning any health program. In the event you use any of the information in this book for yourself, the author and the publisher assume no responsibility for your actions.

For permission to reprint portions of this content or bulk purchases, contact Allison@AllisonMcCuneDavis.com

Author Photograph by: Meggan Whitsitt
Published by Niche Pressworks; NichePressworks.com
Indianapolis, IN

ISBN
Hardcover: 978-1-962956-35-2
Paperback: 978-1-962956-34-5
eBook: 978-1-962956-36-9

Library of Congress Cataloging-in-Publication Data on File at lccn.loc.gov

To my husband, Matthew, my rock, the flagpole to my flag, the guy that has so easily seen to the freedom I needed to pursue my dreams — I love you. And to my five children, Emma, Meg, Henry, Luke, and Sally — what an honor it has been to raise you; you and your dad are the best part of my life. Pursue your dreams and fly high! Always seek God and know He put those dreams inside you.

Table of Contents

Download Your
REIGNITE! SIXTY-DAY DARE TOOLKIT

PACKED WITH MORE RESOURCES AND TOOLS TO STAY ON TRACK!

Go to the link below for:

- Tips on dealing with stress and sleep
- Favorite podcasts and books
- Affirmations for various purposes
- Favorite products and sources
- My basic protocol when pushing through a cold or flu
- The Sixty-Day Dare Group Program
- And more!

These will help you with your Sixty-Day Dare and life in general.

HERE'S TO YOUR LONGEVITY! SPIRIT, SOUL & BODY!
—Allison

AllisonMcCuneDavis.com/Toolkit

PART ONE

MAKING A NEW START

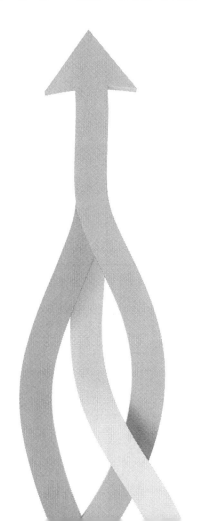

CHAPTER 1

Turning Sixty

It takes a very long time to become young.
— **PABLO PICASSO**

A Big Birthday

It's late afternoon on a chilly day in the fall of 2020 as I pull into my driveway in this behemoth of a twelve-seat, brown Nissan van that the kids call Chewbacca. I like to linger in the driveway for a while with my car still idling. It's my moment for introvert restoration. Secluded. Quiet. Safe.

I notice that the ache in the arch of my foot from the Pilates reformer strap is finally better after taking months to heal. I also recognize that various aches and pains take longer to get better these days. Thankfully, though, I finally prioritized exercise five years ago after decades of ignoring it. I was so worried it was too late but found out — thank you, God — that it wasn't.

I check my phone for various emails, messages, and interesting social media posts before going inside to meet the flurry of activity. Don't all moms do this? Before I get out, I glance in the mirror of my sun visor and notice that the lines in my face are still there. Dang. It's funny how there is always this weird hope that they won't be. With both hands pressed to my cheeks, I slide the skin back toward my ears for the millionth time.

The house will be full when I head inside. All seven of us are back home from the day. These days won't last long, though — soon, the nest will thin out. Our two oldest children will be out of the house any day now (the first job after college for one and going off to college for the other), and the younger three are quite independent.

Finally, my mind turns to the thing I've been trying not to think too much about.

This is the week I turn sixty.

What in the whole, entire world? I mean... I don't even know what to say. How did this happen? I'm ten years from seventy? Twenty years from eighty? Is this it? Am I on a downhill slide? Is there more, or have I already experienced the best years of my life? So many thoughts fly through my mind.

I'm restless. I feel things are about to shift. Decade birthdays have always been times when I asked big questions, and the answers were generally right there. This one is different. I can feel my purpose is morphing somehow. I sense this is a time I may have to do some new things to get me wherever I'm going, even though I may not know exactly why.

Several weeks ago, I decided to take my two youngest and celebrate with a lifelong friend by spending a long weekend at *the beach. My husband has a very full plate, so he can't go, but he is happy to see me able to go. The beach is an antidote whenever I need rejuvenation, answers, or just time and space. It's a tonic for my soul. The trip is only a few days away now.*

I'll try to get a handle on these thoughts then, I promise myself. Feeling better, I turn off the engine and head into the house to greet my family.

A New Way to Plan

During my birthday trip, I keep my promise to myself. It pays off as I find the first of several puzzle pieces that will ultimately spur me into a new direction.

Every morning during the trip, I get up, grab my straw hat and cover-up, and make my way barefoot down to the beach. Walking that slanted, wet, sandy path along the water, I check out each condo and house, wondering who lives there. Smelling that beach air, I let the cool saltwater splash up around my ankles as I walk. Mmmmm. So good.

Then, I head back to the condo and spend the mornings on the couch by the window looking out at the gorgeous green and blue gulf, just thinking, reading, researching things on my laptop, needlepointing, saying a quick prayer here and there.

One day, while on my laptop searching for information, I see an online ad for Jesse Itzler's three-by-four-foot calendar to hang on the wall where you plan your entire year. However, this calendar is different from others. It requires you to FIRST prioritize your special personal and family days and weeks, then add in the rest. This is about living with no regrets. It speaks to my soul. I note that it includes an online community too.[1]

I also love it because I have always been a planner addict. When I was a TV producer years ago, planning was a critical skill. As a homeschooling mom of five, again, I found it paramount.

A significant part of this calendar is the main component, called a Misogi. "Misogi" is a Japanese word for "life-changing event." The calendar requires us to do one thing each year that will transform our lives. Wow! Sounds exciting!

We head back to our small-town home in northwestern Oklahoma. The calendar is my injection of a little something new — at least for this next year. This is not the revelation I am looking for to take me through the next decade by any means, but I can feel it is a first step to something, and I know I need to do it. You know that feeling?

Choosing a Misogi

For the next several months, I contemplate what to choose for my Misogi. I watch many in the online group crush goals, discuss them in detail, and seem to really live life. One day, someone says they are starting this thing called "75 Hard" and asks whether anyone wants to do it with them.

Oh my gosh! Four months earlier, I had come across 75 Hard and listened to the podcast explaining the concept. It's a tough mental and physical challenge created by Andy Frisella, a big, muscular, tattoo-covered guy. The program involves various components, including exercise, diet, and reading for 75 days straight.[2]

When I first saw it, I thought, "There is no way IN THE WORLD, AT ALL, that I can do that. I am NOT his target market." Doing anything for 75 days in a row and not missing a single day sounded nearly impossible, so I quickly put the idea out of my mind.

Now, after watching all these others achieving such huge things, I wonder.

Can I?

I listen to the podcast episode again and spend the next hour mentally sorting out whether I can accomplish this. I normally do a 40-minute Pilates class three to five times a week and walk every now and then. Between those two and some occasional yoga, I think I could tackle the fitness part.

I suddenly realize I CAN do this. It will require every bit of commitment inside me, but it can be my Misogi. I just turned 60, and I'm trying to figure out my life now. I definitely think those things will carry me through.

People Make a Difference

What changed my attitude from believing there was no way I could do it to being willing to commit?

The difference came from being in that online group, seeing other people who were doing big things in their lives.

Motivational speaker Jim Rohn has a saying I've repeated to my kids and friends for many years: "We are the five people we hang out with." Man, there is nothing truer. Those five people had better be people who inspire us and whom we respect, admire, and want to emulate.

The truth behind this saying has to be what changed my mind.

In addition to being in this calendar group full of people doing great things, I was also in Shauna VanBogart's women's online course where, weekly, we asked big questions, assessed our lives, analyzed, got feedback, and tried to pare things down in our lives to the most important.

Plus, I was listening to lots of podcasts and audiobooks about topics like living with a monk or a navy seal for a month, facing all your fears every day for a year (that sounds awful!), and, of course, my usual go-to's: natural health, purpose, and longevity.

Watching and listening to these people do all these challenging things inspired me to get out of my comfort zone and challenge myself too. I was ready to take the plunge and be like them.

> *Watching and listening to these people do all these challenging things inspired me to get out of my comfort zone and challenge myself too.*

75 Hard: Definitely Hard!

Day 1: I am pumped. I've decided to do this crazy thing on the last day of my 25th wedding anniversary trip (to the beach again, of course) with my husband. It's gonna be amazing!

Day 4: It's 2 a.m., and I am half-sleepwalking to the bathroom to pee for the third time tonight. Why? Well, at 11 p.m., I realized I hadn't gotten my water quota in for the day and had to chug 40 ounces. Ugh. Yep, this is hard.

Earlier that day, I was already worrying about finding more people besides my husband to walk with me — thank goodness he's doing the program too! Plus, I need more inspiration than just my podcasts. Gotta call some friends. Also, gotta keep reminding myself this is really good for me. Oh — and yeah, I've gotta figure out how to drink a gallon of water a day before 11 p.m.

As I flop back into bed, my mind drifts back 20 years to something that happened to my father. A brilliant surgeon, he was loved by the whole community, and he absolutely lived his purpose daily, saving lives. Cancer, gunshot wounds, knife fights, car wrecks, aneurysms, anything thoracic-oriented.

On a Monday morning, he was his usual self, feeling good enough to do an appendectomy. However, the next day, one of his doctor friends took a long look at him and said, "Hey, Al, you don't look good. Come see me tomorrow." By Friday, my dad was on the operating table himself. His surgeon was his good friend and colleague; the nurses were people my father had worked with for 30 years.

Late that afternoon, we learned the prognosis: stage 4, inoperable colon cancer. The cancer was so entangled in every part of his gut that there was no way to surgically remove it.

When my father woke up in his hospital bed and learned the truth, everything changed. This big, strong man I had always looked up to —normally so calm — looked at me with confusion and disbelief in his eyes.

"I thought I was bulletproof," he said.

Immediately, I said right back, "I thought you were too."

It felt surreal. How could this leader-of-our-family, pillar-of-the-community father, whom I respected so much, be lying in this bed with this horrible prognosis? It wasn't possible. This wasn't supposed to happen in our family. I couldn't wrap my brain around it. He was supposed to be there for another 20 years at least. I felt weak and couldn't quite catch my breath as I and everyone else grappled with this new truth.

My mind returns to Day 4 of 75 Hard. Heavy sigh. What if my father had just made a few changes in his life a decade or so before that day? We'll never know... but I'm glad I'm doing this. It might not make me bulletproof, but it will definitely help me.

It's hard, but I WILL keep going.

Day 17, 6:30 a.m.: *It's still hard, haha. I shouldn't be surprised since "hard" is part of the title.*

My eyes slowly open, and I see the grey morning light starting to shine through the shutters and reflect off of the big, pink water bottle next to my bed.

My bed feels so warm and soft; I want to stay here for many more hours, especially when I hear rain outside. Hmmm. Rain or not, I have to figure out when I'm going to walk today. I don't have a choice — one of the mandatory two rounds of exercise has to be outside, no matter the weather.

I also have to start my morning water routine — part of the answer to my water-drinking problem. I've learned to drink a lot of water at three particular times: when I wake up and after each of the two rounds of exercise. That, plus always having a water bottle with me, works great to get the gallon in. One thing is a little easier now, at least.

I struggle to untangle from my covers and reach for the water. My weather app says the rain will get worse throughout the day, so I'd better get my butt up now and walk. I throw on my workout clothes, hat, and the raincoat I bought for just this purpose and head out to the street for the 45-minute circuit.

I'm walking in the rain. This is kinda crazy, and I would not be doing it had I not committed. Yet here I am! And ya know, it's not that bad, partly because I know it's my Misogi.

Day 36: *It's the weekend of my husband's employee retreat. Lots of food, drinks, desserts. Ugh. How can I not partake? I've got to plan for this one!*

I eat something from my food plan before I get there so I'm not hungry or tempted when I arrive. I also need to psyche myself up before going into these social gatherings. "Stay the course. You've gone this far," I reassure myself.

The bad news is that though I make it through the day without going off the food plan, by 10 p.m., I still have a quart of water to drink. Dang it. The day got away from me, and either I drink it now and get up multiple times to go the bathroom, or I start the whole damn thing over.

I chug the water. And as the weeks have gone on, I've noticed something: I feel much more focused. I have stronger boundaries and can simply say no to things that will get in the way of accomplishing my 75 Hard tasks for the day. I am developing the mental toughness Andy Frisella talks about as part of the program. It is getting a tiny bit easier. And I am absolutely not starting over.

Day 55: *This routine is becoming just that — routine. It's my new normal. My digestive system is working really well. The weird spots on my face have disappeared. I know from my health studies that our skin reflects the gut. That means good things must be happening there.*

"Stay attentive," I tell myself. They say people get lax after a while. If I miss one item on any day, I start over — no exceptions. If I finish, I can order a cool medallion. I have done this for 55 days now, and I only have 20 more to go. The longer I go, the more I have to lose. It would be totally and completely horrible if I messed this up now. And I want that dang medallion.

Day 75: YES!!! I did it! I have done the full 75 days. I've lost 12 pounds. And I've created some better habits.

It has definitely changed my life mentally. I can't believe I did it! I'm not sure I've ever done anything as challenging. I am thrilled and ecstatic and so proud of myself! Good job, girlfriend! I hop on the computer and order the medallion immediately.

Today, three years later, the medallion still sits right next to the keyboard of my computer. I pick it up and turn it over in my hand all the time and think, "I did that." Such a great reminder that if I really set my mind to do something, I can. Wow!

Why I Wrote This Book

I don't do the five 75 Hard tasks every single day now, but I sure do a lot better than I used to. And yet, even after that accomplishment, I wanted more. The question still remained: What will I do next, for the long term? What can I sink my teeth into that will help others? I was still restless.

A few weeks later, I headed to Dallas to hang out with my childhood friend of fifty-some years. She had turned sixty just a month prior. We met for drinks with several of her friends who are in our age range. We eventually started talking about that fact, and she laughingly said, "Well, I hear sixty is the gateway to old age."

I felt a visceral response, like I had been punched in the gut. "No! I do not accept that!" My voice was vehement. Then, I laughed. She laughed. But man, I meant it.

Her statement continued to haunt me. On my walk with my husband the next morning, I told him about the conversation, my voice fervent with the same passion. Two weeks later, on the morning of July 4th, I was lying in bed, doing my favorite meditative breathing exercise. In the midst of it, and in a flash, I knew exactly what I had to do.

I have to write a book.

What? I thought, surprised.

Then, it suddenly seemed so clear. Well, of course. I have to write a book!

This is always how it happens. After months and months of searching and struggle and restlessness and seeking and praying, in a simple moment, with no advance warning, it all becomes clear. You know exactly what you have to do. It's crazy. Sometimes, it takes so much patience to wait for those moments to come.

The Self-Perpetuating Circle of Purpose

They say that your passion or purpose can be born out of the things that break your heart, make you angry, or create an intense emotional response. That is definitely true for me.

That morning, it all came together. I realized my long-held desire was to combine everything I have studied and loved all these years into a system. The natural health, personal development, spiritual seeking, new-habit-forming, longevity-oriented, goal-setting, planning-my-life techniques into a process that is easily doable, easily understandable, and moves the needle forward for you in your life in all of the important areas. Though it's a baby-step method, it creates results. That's what this book is meant to give you. Results.

This is the path to finding good health, passion, purpose, and a plan for your life. It involves a framework I call The Self-Perpetuating Circle of Purpose. I'll go into that more in the next chapter.

The great news is that these things go right along with principles of longevity — one of my favorite subjects!

We All Need Guides

On this quest involving the calendar, 75 Hard, the online course, the books, and even the exercise routine I'd started five years prior, it became very evident to me that I needed help. I needed a guide. I needed someone to assist me in finding the next steps quicker than I could on my own.

I've had so many guides and mentors along the way. I couldn't help but realize that if I needed one, then others probably would, too. There were probably others around sixty out there trying to figure out what to do with their lives like I was. If I could give them help, tips, or new ideas, that would be a jump start so they wouldn't have to look so hard for the answers. That's partly what I hope to do for you in this book — but it's also more.

This Book Is Made for YOUR New Start

As I thought more about what I wanted to do with this book, I realized it would be helpful to create a plan anyone can use to start working within the framework of the Self-Perpetuating Circle of Purpose and learn more about their own health needs.

This plan is called the **Sixty-Day Dare**. It combines all of the elements of longevity in the areas of the body, the brain, and the world — everything that makes your life worth living. It's also flexible, allowing you to design your own plan within some general parameters.

It is meant to help you unlock more knowledge, skills, and habits for thriving in this phase of your life and possibly even assist you in discovering a whole new purpose.

Why Sixty?

According to neuroscientist Dr. Caroline Leaf, it takes two to eight months to create a new habit, depending on the situation[3], so I've started with sixty days. Also, sixty is around the age when many women make transformational changes for the next few decades of life. It certainly was for me. It all makes a nice kind of sense.

This really IS a START. It doesn't end after sixty days. You'll be able to keep employing these Sixty-Day Dare cycles, adding new elements to up-level your life a step at a time.

You can do this on your own, or if you'd like help, you are welcome to join our Sixty-Day Dare program. Details are in the *Reignite!* toolkit, which you can find out how to get at the end of the book.

Are You Ready?

How are you feeling about your current situation? How about the future?

How do you feel? Are you healthy? Does your body feel good enough to do the things you want to do?

Are you restless? Are you looking for something that will make you wake up with a smile on your face and excitement for the day?

Are you at the end of raising your children? Are they out of the house? Maybe some are still living at home?

What will you do for the next decade? The next twenty years? How will you spend your time?

Are your daily activities exactly what you want them to be? Are you too busy? Not involved enough?

Are you listening to your brain's negative self-talk? Do you have more moments of anxiety, depression, or loneliness than you'd like?

What do you desire deep, deep down? So deep you might be afraid to even voice?

Based on your daily routines, will your life lead to good mental awareness and physical health in the long run?

Will you be able to have joyful experiences with your children and grandchildren, and maybe even great-grandchildren?

Will you be able to go on trips with your loved ones, have fun holiday dinners together, go on long walks, and experience nature and our beautiful world?

Will you be cognitively capable enough to advise your children when they come to you with their family's or children's troubles? Or maybe just to have a deep conversation?

Will you be able to rock your grandchildren to sleep or be counted on to watch them for an evening or a weekend?

Will you be able to easily travel — whether around your state, your country, or the world?

Are you on track to live a full, satisfying, well-lived life?

If any of these things are on your mind, then read on.

CHAPTER 2

Starting Down This Path

Your body holds deep wisdom. Trust in it. Learn from it.
Nourish it. Watch your life transform and be healthy.
— **ERIN KEANE**

Rachel, 25 and a stay-at-home mom, is at the hospital emergency room with her infant son *AGAIN*. They've been in and out of the ER every few weeks over the past six months.

She holds her baby, feeling helpless, while he squirms and screams, grabbing his ear. She feels his head again. The fever seems to be dissipating since she gave him the baby Tylenol.

"Why is this happening? What am I doing wrong?" she thinks.

Another new doctor walks back into the room. "He has an ear infection again," he says, handing her a prescription. "Give him this antibiotic, and that will do the trick. You're also going to have to tell your mother she cannot smoke around your son anymore. This is adding to the problem."

Rachel shakes her head. "All these different doctors, and I'm just now hearing this about the smoking?" she thinks. "Oh, my goodness, how will I tell my mom? She is not going to be happy. She may not come over anymore. But all of these drugs cannot be good for him, either. I have to tell her."

She prays, "Dear God, after this, if he gets sick again, I'm not going to put him on antibiotics, but I don't know what to do. Please show me what to do."

The following week, she learns from a church friend that a naturopath occasionally teaches moms in town. Rachel goes to the next class and asks what to do for her son's ear infections.

"Get garlic ear drops," the naturopath says. "One to two drops in each ear with a cotton ball. Follow it up a few times, and he'll be fine."

Two days later, Rachel and her son visit her mom, who is, of course, smoking. Rachel doesn't feel comfortable asking her mother not to smoke in her own house; she was offended enough when asked not to smoke in Rachel's.

Thankfully, Rachel has a plan if her son gets sick.

Two days later, like clockwork, her son spikes a 103 temperature and is crying and screaming in pain. However, within 20 minutes after Rachel applies the ear drops, his pain and fever begin to subside.

She can't believe it! After continuing for a few days, the ear issue appears to be gone. Thrilled and relieved, Rachel feels like such a better mom now. Her intuition and prayer led her to answers.

A paradigm shift and a path into natural health begins. The experience has motivated her to investigate herbs and tinctures, homeopathy, and apple cider vinegar, to name a few remedies, for herself and her family.

Quite a few years later, Rachel, now a single mom of six, moves to town and starts looking for community. She begins attending a monthly natural health class that I lead. She learns more about nutrition, supplements, herbs, essential oils (the more potent blood of the plant), and good self-care — certainly what a single mom of six needs!

And her journey doesn't only include physical health. Over time, she begins working on her relationships, childhood issues, divorce baggage, and emotional health. Counseling, journaling, prayer, and connecting emotional root causes to physical ailments are a few techniques Rachel uses to understand who she is. The emotions are complicated, but she has the fortitude to address them little by little.

Eventually, feeling more settled, Rachel starts to study the healing power of plants. When she makes the connection that God put the plants on earth for our health, she is inspired to study their chemical constituents and how they affect the body. The revelations bring another paradigm shift in her life.

She attends a demonstration class on Raindrop Technique®, an immune-boosting massage that involves highly antibacterial and antiviral essential oils like oregano and thyme, reflexology on the spinal points of the feet, and specific massage techniques on the back and spine.[4] She is inspired and continues to study.

Today, Rachel is remarried to a wonderful man, and her children are almost all grown and gone. She has a business in which she uses Raindrop Technique® to help people improve their own health.

She loves the people who come to see her, is invested in them, and wants to see them heal. She also teaches classes about natural health. She sees these activities as her purpose and ministry in the world now.

Finding a Better Way

Rachel's journey started when she realized she didn't know everything she could do for her children and herself. She had to do her own research and learn from other sources instead of just taking for granted that healthcare professionals were giving her the best advice and there was nothing else out there.

This applies not only to Rachel but to anyone. While not everyone who discovers natural healing goes on to become a practitioner like Rachel, anyone can up-level the health of their own lives in all the key areas. It just takes a little knowledge and some practice.

So, How Do We Get That?

One day, I was staring at the huge whiteboard in my office, thinking about how I could simplify the road to good health and longevity for you to be able to grasp and engage in. Something you would actually do. "God, what is it?" I muttered.

This circle popped up in my mind, with three sections and then the words "Self-Perpetuating Circle of Purpose." It was definitely a God moment.

Self-Perpetuating Circle of Purpose

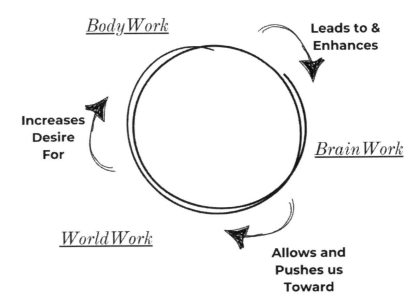

Figure 2.1 The Self-Perpetuating Circle of Purpose revolves around the three principles of health and longevity: BodyWork, BrainWork, and WorldWork. They are interrelated and work to support each other.

This circle revolves around three principles of health and longevity: BodyWork, BrainWork, and WorldWork. They are interrelated and work to support each other. We'll talk a lot more about that in the book.

Physical issues, whether yours or maybe your child's, usually take priority because of pain or suffering of some sort. These are within the BodyWork aspect. Sorting out mental or emotional issues — BrainWork — can come next once we have the physical fortitude for it. Or, we do sometimes have to start there if mental issues are prevalent — and most times, attacking the emotional issue with physical solutions helps tremendously. And, when we are balanced in our mental and physical health, we are able to really use our gifts for the world. This is the ultimate fulfillment. WorldWork reinforces and energizes the others. These three areas continually overlap, and as we get better in any of them, we raise our bar.

How I Created This Framework

This framework is built from my years of working with women, my family, my own health journey, and much investigation into natural health, longevity, the brain, and the body. Obviously, I can't include everything, but here are just a few of my favorite researchers who traveled the world in search of truth.

Dr. Weston A. Price

Weston A. Price, a dentist, researched isolated groups of people in the 1920s and 30s across the world. He found a correlation between the time when processed food made a strong entrance into the American grocery store and home and changes in patients' teeth and jaw formation.[5] He was one of the researchers who wrote about the healing qualities of raw milk, as well as fermented and nutrient-dense foods.

Jordan Rubin

When Crohn's disease threatened to take the life of Jordan Rubin, now a natural health expert in the United States, he and his parents searched the world for traditional medical answers. Finding none, they turned to alternative medicine and eventually found solutions, which he documented in his book called *The Maker's Diet.*[6]

Dr. William Davis

Dr. William Davis, a cardiologist, traveled the world to figure out why wheat in America had become so bad. He took all his heart patients off of it and saw dramatic healing.[7] According to his research, it certainly isn't the waving grains of wheat from yesteryear. However, take heart, there is good wheat available. You just have to find it. (My *Reignite!* Toolkit lists resources — see the end of the book.)

Dr. D. Gary Young

Dr. D. Gary Young is known as the father of the modern-day essential oils movement. Dr. Young did two very significant things.

First, he rediscovered the benefits of high-grade essential oils to the body for physical, emotional, mental, and spiritual health. Essential oils were the medicines of the previous hundreds and thousands of years, even going back to biblical times with frankincense and myrrh. They can be inhaled into the limbic system, the center of memory, emotions, and trauma. They can be applied topically for things like burns and wound care or taken internally for other health benefits. Understanding these different effects is just the beginning.[8] He also developed supplements infused with essential oils that were shown to be absorbed more quickly and more fully into the body. To control the growth of these plants in virgin soils, along with cultivation and distillation, he started or acquired farms all over the world.

Second, he spent the 1980s searching for the longest-lived people — those who lived more than a hundred years and were relatively healthy. He found one such group in Ningxia, China, who attributed their long lives to consuming three things in this order: the Ningxia wolfberry (one specific variety of seventeen), ginseng, and green tea.[9] (As an aside, I've been drinking two to six ounces of that wolfberry puree/juice daily for over a dozen years and can attest to its wonder.)

Dan Buettner

Twenty years later, in the early 2000s, Dan Buettner, National Geographic writer, explorer, and author of the book *The Blue Zones*,"[10] was also investigating long-lived people. Ultimately, he and several other demographers identified five locations around the world that also had large groups of centenarians — those who've lived at least a hundred years and were living long, healthy lives. The sites are in Sardinia, Italy; Okinawa, Japan; Ikaria, Greece; Loma Linda, California; and the Nicoya peninsula of Costa Rica.

After years of studying these groups, they came up with the lifestyle principles[11] the centenarians in these locations have in common. You'll read more about this and other longevity studies in the next chapter.

"Too Old" Is a Myth

If you think the centenarians studied by world explorers are just unicorns, and this kind of life isn't possible for "normal people," you've fallen for the myth that, at some point, you're "too old" to change, improve your life, or do the thing that "only younger people do."

I know a little bit about the myth of "Too Old." I've been defying it for quite some time. I married at 35. First baby at 37 by C-section (and told it was a geriatric pregnancy. That's hysterical.). Second baby at age 40, at home. Third baby at age 42, also at home. Fourth baby adopted from Russia at 46. Fifth baby adopted from Ethiopia at 50. Starting to exercise regularly at 55. Writing a book at 60.

And there are so many others who have pursued their dreams much later than I.

One wonderful example is Instagram-based fitness influencer Joan MacDonald. I love following her. She is 78 and started getting in shape with the help of her health-coach daughter when she was 70 after her doctor wanted to put her on more medications. Now she is in fantastic muscular shape and is followed by almost two million people. She is an inspiration.

Busting the "Too Old" Myth Wide Open

If you think the "too old" argument is solid, think again. Here's proof:

- American artist Grandma Moses started painting at 76.[12]
- Chef Julia Child wrote her first cookbook at fifty.[13]
- Laura Ingalls Wilder finally got her first book, *Little House in the Big Woods*, published when she was 65.[14]
- Colonel Harland Sanders started Kentucky Fried Chicken at 65 after being broke.[15]
- Mommy Choi was 70 when she discovered cooking as her hobby. She sells her Korean-inspired sauces online and in stores.[16]
- Jane Fonda and Lily Tomlin did seven seasons of their TV show *Grace and Frankie*, ending at the ages of 84 and 82.[17]
- Mathea Allansmith, 92, is the oldest woman to run a marathon.[18]
- Nola Ochs went back to college and graduated at 95.[19]

The Sixty-Day Dare: A Plan to Start the Circle

In the Sixty-Day Dare, you'll get a choice of things to do daily in each of the three major categories — there are five choices (which I call the "Big Five") in each category. Your job is to pick one item per category.

If you challenge yourself, committing to and engaging in these activities for sixty days will be life-changing. Until we start changing our daily habits, including both behavioral and thought-based habits, our lives won't change. Remember this essential principle:

Our future is hidden in our daily routine.
— **MIKE MURDOCK**

This plan will work — but only if you commit to it. It will give you a clear path up front so you don't have to spend a lot of time figuring out each day what you need to do; you will have already made all your decisions and can just start achieving the goals.

Be Your Own Health Detective

As with Rachel, when you become your own health detective, you find that taking charge of your health is a defining moment of change. With the technology at our fingertips today, there is no excuse for this not to happen.

When you become your own health detective, you find that taking charge of your health is a defining moment of change.

Also, understand that this book isn't meant to take care of everything for you. It's meant to give you a framework to work within to make good decisions and develop healthy habits.

The gap between traditional, ancient medicines and the world of modern medicine that rules Western society is wide, but it is ever so slowly closing. Understanding this is important as you advocate for your health and that of your loved ones.

Thankfully, practitioners such as naturopaths, functional or integrative medical doctors, chiropractors, and others are bridging the gap. Because of these kinds of doctors, the old Thomas Edison quote is very slowly coming to fruition: "The doctor of the future will give no medicine but will interest the patient in the care of the human frame, in diet, and in the cause and prevention of disease."

And while preventative medicine (the word "medicine" comes from the Latin root, *mederi*, which means "to heal") is crucial, at the same time, we still thank God for emergency medicine, surgeries that save lives, and scientific discoveries that benefit us all.

This book is a beginning. Whether you already know about alternative medicine or not, if you take the dare and start down this path with a commitment to all three areas, you will absolutely transform your life. You've probably heard the saying, "when your health is good, you don't ever think about it, but when it's not, it's the only thing you think about." Our goal is to think about lots of other things!

Start where you are. Use what you have. Do what you can.
— ARTHUR ASHE

Self-Evaluation: What's Your Current Status?

Let's do a quick self-evaluation to look at where you are in key areas of your life right now.

Give each of these categories a score of 1 to 10, in which 10 would be the best it could ever be, and 1 would be the worst. Be honest. Go with your gut feeling for each item. This is just for your eyes. No one else needs to see it.

_____ **Food:** Do you eat mostly healthy foods?

_____ **Supplements:** Are you taking any or do you know if you're taking the right ones?

_____ **Water:** Do you drink ½ your body weight in ounces of water daily?

_____ **Exercise:** Do you exercise daily?

_____ **Sleep:** Do you sleep at least seven to nine hours a night?

_____ **Mental Development:** How stressed are you?

_____ **Personal Development:** Do you know yourself well?

_____ **Spiritual Development:** Do you give this attention?

_____ **Family Relationships:** How are they?

_____ **Romantic Relationship:** How is this?

_____ **Friendships:** Do you have satisfying friendships?

_____ **Purpose/Career/Mission:** Do you know yours?

_____ **Finances:** Are they in good shape?

_____ **Fun/Restoration/Hobbies:** Do you spend time on these?

_____ **Environment (Home, car, office, etc.):** Are the areas you spend the most time in neat, organized, beautiful, and devoid of toxins?

Now, take a look. What area or areas did you rate the lowest? Keep those in mind because they may be key areas that you will want to work on in your first Sixty-Day Dare.

Oh, and just an aside: If you are not in a romantic relationship and you like it that way, then give yourself a high score. Not everyone needs to be in one.

Now, Where Do You Want to Be?

I wrote this book to not just tell you but SHOW you that no matter what your life looks like, you can change it.

Everyone has his or her own threshold. Everyone has that moment when they are sick of hearing their own excuses and justifications, sick of not fulfilling promises to themselves, sick of being overweight and out of shape, sick of starting something umpteen million times only to quit a few weeks or months down the road. That does not have to be you.

This book isn't about starting some new fad diet or program. It's about finding that new thing, that beautiful reason to get up in the morning and fulfill a new purpose that everything leading up to now has been preparing you for, just as it did for every previous purpose. It's also about learning to live a naturally healthy life, feeling good, and having the energy you need to do all you want.

When you look again at the areas you evaluated, maybe there are some you think are not ideal.

Think about who and where you want to be in a year, in five years, in ten years. Think big. Now, write these answers down in your journal or notebook. How do you feel looking at them? Will they take you out of your comfort zone? That's a good sign.

If you feel like they're impossible, that's probably not true. You have the ability to get there. All you need is to believe you are capable and start taking some baby steps to get there. Let's erase those doubts and get going, my dear! You've got this!

CHAPTER 3

It's Hard to Be Healthy, But Solutions Exist

If it doesn't challenge you, it won't change you.
— FRED DEVITO

A New Way

It's a hot summer day in 1994 Sherman Oaks, California. I'm 33 years old. I'm chatting with my new neighbor by the little pool in our small eight-plex apartment building to which I recently moved. She is about ten years older than me and very "California" with her flowing caftans and herbs and plants and various weird bottles of potions on her kitchen counter that I can see through her sliding glass door.

Hesitantly, I tell her I'm dealing with a yeast infection that has resurfaced multiple times over the years and is extremely aggravating.

She quickly says, "Oh, you must go to my TCM doctor. He will totally help you!"

"TCM?" I ask, not wanting to look ignorant. "What's that?"

"Traditional Chinese Medicine," she answers.

Ha! My surgeon father would flip his lid, but I am intrigued. I've used the medically suggested protocols for years. The infections still come, and I'm sick of them. I've got to try something different, for goodness' sake.

I guess it's a good sign that I have to wait six weeks to see him. When I finally arrive, his office looks like a normal doctor's office but with lots of supplements lined up behind the front desk. Hmmm. Interesting.

In his examining room, he has a large briefcase open on a table with lots of tiny glass vials in it. After we talk a bit about what is going on, he says, "Hold out your right arm, and in your left hand, hold this vial. When I press down on your arm, I want you to resist."

What the hell?

Ok. Whatever.

We do this with lots of different vials. Sometimes, I could resist fine, and other times, my arm would go weak. This is my first experience with Muscle Response Testing (MRT).

The substances in the vials are all kinds of things, including foods and common allergens. He is testing to see what makes my body weak. Afterward, he tells me to cut out dairy completely, possibly for a year. I might be able to add it back in *later. I realize I eat dairy at almost all my meals. Homogenized and pasteurized milk with cereal, pastas and cheese, cheese and crackers, and the list goes on. He also gives me some herbs to take for a few months.*

This is my first experience with herbs and solutions that are radically different from the medicines I grew up with. So is the idea that treatments could include something besides prescriptions and over-the-counter drugs.

This is the moment I learn that herbs — plants — can assist in healing and that our bodies are actually made to heal if we can just support them in the right way, if we can stop putting the wrong foods and fake, synthetic concoctions made in a lab into our precious, organic life form made by God.

Cars must have the exact right fuel. We probably should, too. People instinctively ate correctly for thousands of years. Why have we forgotten?

I learned then that we shouldn't just bandage a symptom. We need to get to the root of an issue and heal it. From that day on, I start to change the way I eat. I also take the herbs and continue on down this path from where it started, there, in his office.

In 30 years, I have never gotten another yeast infection, and trust me, I haven't been perfect — far from it. However, I am much more cognizant of what I put in or on my body.

It Isn't Easy

It's hard to be healthy in the Western world. Don't feel bad if you think you haven't done a good job in this department. You and I have grown up in a modern world with a "chemistry is best," "processed food is convenient," and "pills fix everything" mentality. Most of our parents and some grandparents were living in that same world, and we just learned it from them.

Heck, I grew up on bologna and mustard sandwiches, bright white bread, jiggly gelatin cubes full of red dye 40, and canned green beans. I bet you did, too. I had an awesome mom, but she grew up in the 50s and had her four children in the 60s, smack-dab in the middle of marketing schemes by food companies showing how "the modern housewife's job could be so much easier and the results just as good as always." She was just following their advice.

One rebellious thing she did was to breastfeed all four of her children, which was rare at this time. By 1971, only 25 percent of women were breastfeeding their babies. The decline began in the 1920s with the advent of the refrigerator. It could store this new thing called "formula." This is a perfect illustration of just one avenue where marketing convinced moms that the recipes of science, Big Pharma, and big food were better than Mother Nature. Breastfeeding didn't make a comeback until the 1970s. La Leche League tells us the stats: "... in 1970, the percentage of American babies breastfed *at all* stood at around 27 percent; in 1990, around 52 percent; and in 2007, around 76 percent."[20]

Don't even get me started on the toxic ingredients that the United States allows in everything from housecleaning products to makeup, skincare, shampoo, toothpaste, laundry soap, and the list goes on and on and on.

The EWG (Environmental Working Group) tells us the U.S. lags behind 80 other countries, including the EU, who "have restricted or completely banned more than 1600 chemicals from cosmetic products. By contrast, the U.S. FDA has banned or restricted only nine chemicals for safety reasons."[21] Read Dr. Casey Means new book, *Good Energy*, to dive deep into this and similar topics.[22]

We must, very, very intentionally, break out of this matrix to see clearly. I like to look at most situations and ask myself, "What did God intend? What would the natural way be in this situation?" Those questions help me get to answers that I hope are in the right direction. Each of us truly must have a paradigm shift in our mindset and our habits in the face of American culture. Again, it is not easy to be healthy, but it is possible. You just need a plan.

> *Each of us truly must have a paradigm shift in our mindset and our habits in the face of American culture.*

How Did We Get to This Situation?

This subject is complicated and involves many aspects. Entire books are written on it, so this will be a very cursory overview.

Don't get too depressed. Things will get better! We have to talk about the bad, and then we will get to the good!

The World of Medicine

Significant changes began in the early 1900's when a guy named Abraham Flexner was tasked by John D. Rockefeller, Andrew Carnegie, and others to create a report on the state of medical education in the United States. He was to help align it more with German education methods, lab research, and patented medicine. Congress affirmed the report. According to a Pub Med paper from the NIH Natural Library of Medicine:

> [Flexner] advocated for the closing of nearly 80 percent of all the contemporary programs in homeopathy, naturopathy, eclectic therapy, physical therapy, osteopathy, and chiropractic. Very few institutions (approximately 20 percent of those mentioned in his report) were subsequently able to comply with Flexner's constraints and prescriptions, while most had to shut their doors forever, particularly those in the already medically underserved large rural areas of the American Midwest and the Southern States.[23]

Add to this that Rockefeller realized he could use the by-products of his oil production in patented medicines. Hmmm, that doesn't sound good. Also, Rockefeller did much funding of medical schools around the country. Hmmm.

The conflicts of interest seem to abound here. Now, over a century later, there is much to sort through to understand how we got where we are today. Questioning medical authorities is frowned upon, but honestly, at this point, we don't have a choice if we want good outcomes. The system has become so convoluted and corrupt it is almost impossible to know what to do.

Dr. Means comments on another issue related to the problem, saying, "We have been gaslighted to not ask questions over the past fifty years at the exact time chronic disease rates have exploded.[24]

Oh my. What a tangled web has been woven.

Listen to your doc for things like a broken bone or an emergency issue that puts your life on the line. For chronic conditions, ask lots of questions, do some research, and don't feel bad about it.

Medical Schools

Only a fifth of medical schools require medical students to take ANY courses on nutrition, even though we have mounds of evidence showing it is a critical component of health.

David Eisenberg, adjunct professor of nutrition at Harvard's T.H. Chan School of Public Health, said, "Today, most medical schools in the United States teach less than 25 hours of nutrition over four years. The fact is less than 20 percent of medical schools have a single required course in nutrition; it's a scandal. It's outrageous. It's obscene."[25]

Once doctors are in the real world, life gets busy. There is little time between patients, hospitals, surgeries, and home life to do one's own research. Pharmaceutical reps make their way into doctor's offices to give them the latest drug information, and the doctors rely upon it. However, no nutritional experts are there explaining food and metabolic pathways and how healing can occur with what nature has provided. In fact, many health professionals regard these people as quacks.

Dr. Means also tells us that when she finished medical school, she had to choose one of forty-two specialties to devote her life to. After five years of training, she could have gone further into a sub-specialty focused on an area of the body only a few inches in diameter.

Wow. You can imagine how one could inevitably not see a holistic view of the body when the doctor is so micro-focused. Why does this person continue to have sinus infections? Should we do surgery or figure out what is going on in the rest of the body? Those questions took her out of a surgical future and into a world of cell metabolism and healing the whole body. I'm thankful for her book.

Big Pharma

Big Pharma consists of privately owned, for-profit drug companies that do large research projects and then create and patent drugs to sell. A key factor to understand is that one cannot patent anything that is natural, a plant for instance. So, obviously, Big Pharma is never motivated to spend large amounts of money to study natural solutions like herbs and plants.

These pharmaceutical products treat symptoms versus getting to the root cause of a problem. They also all have side effects because they are not natural.

Advertising

America and New Zealand are the only countries in the entire world that allow direct-to-consumer advertising of prescription drugs. This began in the mid-1980s in America. The author of *Drugs, Money, & Secret Handshakes*, Robin Feldman, tells us, "... Research shows that advertising medicine to consumers prompts inappropriate prescriptions, increases adverse patient outcomes and boosts drug prices."[26]

Lobbying

Pharmaceutical companies are among the biggest lobbyists in Washington, D.C. The FDA, the government agency that approves drugs for the marketplace, is partially funded by those drug companies. Isn't this a conflict of interest?

Ten years ago, a Washington, D.C., senator from my state told my health freedom activist friend that the Big Pharma machine is too big to change and best to go back home and make a difference in your own community. She did.

Today, activists *are* sounding the alarm and just beginning to be heard in D.C. With stats like these, thank God. Dr. Means is one of them and gives us these statistics:

- 74 percent of American adults are dealing with overweight or obesity.
- 40 percent of children are overweight or suffer from obesity.
- 52 percent of American adults have prediabetes or type 2 diabetes.
- 30 percent of teens have prediabetes (this was 11 percent in 2002).
- 1 in 36 children are on the autism spectrum (up from 1 in 150 in the year 2000).[27]

And the list goes on. Why?

Pharma Studies

I learned recently from John Abramson, MD, who wrote *Sickening: How Big Pharma Broke American Health Care and How We Can Repair It*,[28] drug companies research a drug. They present their data analysis to medical journals like *JAMA* (*Journal of American Medical Association*), where their analysis is peer-reviewed. Doctors relying on these studies then believe the drug is good.

They don't realize the Big Pharma companies do NOT give the raw data to the medical journal or to the peer reviewers. The reviewers must rely on the summaries or very curated data from the drug companies. The complete data might only come to light if, say, five years later, there are bad outcomes and they wind up in court. That is when they would have to present their data.

It is a broken system.

Don't take offense here if you are on some drugs that you believe are saving your life or making you feel better. Again, no judgment! I'm not saying you should get off of any medication. Keep in contact with your doctor, let them know you are making lifestyle changes, and discuss whether that might allow you to lessen what you are taking. Always the necessary disclaimer: This is not medical advice. It is simply education.

And I understand. In fact, I still take a pill for my thyroid, though I am always on the hunt for natural solutions.

The Western Mindset: The Faster, the Better

I know how you think, because I do it too. It has been ingrained in us from the beginning. We want it fast, and we want it now, and we don't want it to take too long. Can you imagine how much worse that thinking has become in our world of smartphones, social media, and the resulting super-short attention spans since the early 2000s?

We stay home and get on our devices rather than making the effort to socialize, invest in friendships, or work on relationships. And all of this affects mental health.

We scroll through our phones at lightning speed, watching 15-second videos for constant dopamine hits. Then, when we have to concentrate or work hard on one thing or even just read a book, it's really hard.

To Make Things Worse...

Our habits don't support our health.

We don't drink enough water, the lack of which creates headaches, sluggish digestion, dull skin, fatigue, and weight gain. Our bodies are 60 percent water, and those supple organs, arteries, and veins need to be hydrated with water, not soda, to stay in good shape.

We don't move our bodies enough because modernity makes everything so easy. Our circadian rhythms are messed up, so sleep is a problem. And the list goes on.

Making things even harder, our food is depleted of nutrients, especially minerals, and is high in toxins because of fertilizers and processing. Good gracious, it's a rough road.

What About Purpose?

Large numbers are unhappy at work. A Gallup study tells us that "In the U.S., 50 percent of workers reported feeling stressed at their jobs on a daily basis, 41 percent as being worried, 22 percent as sad, and 18 percent as angry…. Workers are unhappy at home, at the office, working 30-hour work weeks and 60-hour work weeks."[29] It doesn't seem to matter where they work or for how long.

To see how purpose affects our health in a good way, check out this Pub Med study in the NIH Library of Medicine. It included 13,770 adults who were assessed up to five times across eight years. Those in the top quarter of having purpose in life had a 24 percent lower likelihood of becoming physically inactive, a 33 percent lower likelihood of developing sleep problems, and a 22 percent lower likelihood of developing unhealthy body mass index, in other words, being overweight.[30]

I don't think there is any doubt we should get clear on our purpose in the world, and it needs to make us excited to get up each morning.

The Result: The Self-Limiting Circle of Loss

Let's look at the opposite of the Self-Perpetuating Circle of Purpose and how we can get into a terrible cycle if we don't take serious steps to break out of it.

Self-Limiting Circle of Loss

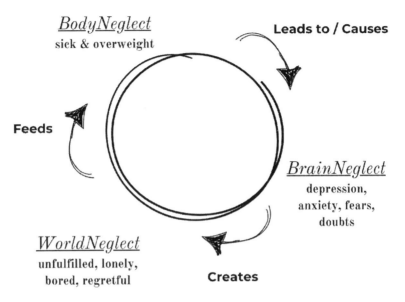

BodyNeglect
sick & overweight

Leads to / Causes

Feeds

BrainNeglect
depression,
anxiety, fears,
doubts

WorldNeglect
unfulfilled, lonely,
bored, regretful

Creates

Figure 3.1 The Self-Limiting Circle of Loss creates a cycle of self-negation, with a process very similar to the Self-Perpetuating Circle of Purpose. In the Circle of Loss, the areas of neglect work together to create destructive patterns in mental/physical health, relationships, and life purpose.

Looking at this cycle, shown in Figure 3.1, you can see how, just as the positive circle's elements we looked at in the previous drawing all reinforce themselves, those in the negative circle all affect the others, too. If you aren't feeling physically well, your illness can affect your mental health. And if your physical and mental health aren't good, you'll feel unable to do things that would fulfill you. Those include working on your world purpose or even just getting out of the house to see family and friends or exercise! Yet

Western medicine seems to only just now be seeing these links. You can be way ahead in that respect.

Be Like Rachel: Take Charge of Your Health

I hate to be the one to say this, but here is the truth most people don't want to acknowledge: No one else is going to really look out for you except you. It is up to each of us to research, to advocate, and to decide what is best for us. That research can definitely include advice from various professionals. However, don't do what they say without your own due diligence unless, of course, your life is on the line at that moment.

Everyone is capable of making positive change — even through tiny steps.

You don't have to decide to run two miles a day and eat only one meal. You could decide to simply walk to the end of the block each day and cut out drinking soda. Start there.

Don't let this negative cycle rule your life. The sooner you break out of it, the better off you'll be.

What We Can Achieve with a Little Effort

Let's go back to take a closer look at the centenarians in the Blue Zones and Ningxia, China. From the research in 2011 into the Blue Zones, Buettner found that "people reach age 100 at ten times greater rates than in the United States."[31] Wow!

Their age doesn't seem to hamper them from still leading fulfilling, happy lives. In all these areas, they take long walks (a good marker of longevity), garden, farm, cook, and do housework. They have extended social dinners and many taking part in the preparation. They have daily rituals to reduce stress and its related inflammation, including prayer, napping, social time with family and friends, and eating to only 80 percent satiety. Yes, I think that last part sounds hard too, but it is important. The brain requires up to thirty minutes to get the message that the stomach is full. We've gotta slow down.

There are no nursing homes in these areas. Families and friends take care of each other, and the younger generations understand the need for the wisdom of their elders. Dr. Liji Thomas, MD, also tells us they have "low rates of cancer, cardiovascular disease, and almost no dementia.... They are sheep farmers, walking at least five miles up and down mountains... They thrive on faith, family and work." [32] Some have been in social support groups since age five.

Why are they so different from older people in Western civilization? Much of it is their environment, which nudges them into healthy behaviors.

What About Genetics?

What we find in most long-lived people is the remarkable evidence demonstrated in the famous Danish Twin study, which took place over the entire 20th century and looked at almost 2900 sets of twins. It shows that in all of the longevity factors, genes contribute to only 24.5 percent. Thus, as they said in the study, "longevity seems to be only moderately heritable." [33] That is great news!

More recently, *Science Daily* reported, "The vast majority of diseases, including many cancers, diabetes, and Alzheimer's disease, have a genetic contribution of

5 to 10 percent at best."[34] Again, fantastic news. Since our environment and our lifestyle choices play crucial roles, we have much more control than we thought or have been told.

We can take it to mean that it's not always special genetics these people have — the secrets are in their environment and what they're doing within it every day. In other words, their habits.

> *It's not always special genetics these people have — the secrets are in their environment and what they're doing within it every day. In other words, their habits.*

Solutions: Healthy Culture and Healthy Habits

How do we get from where we are to a plan that truly supports our health and longevity? In the constant search for what keeps us young and vital, there have been a number of studies over the years on longevity. They all seem to tell us the same things.

There is Dan Buettner, explorer and National Geographic Fellow, and his study on the commonalities of the large groups of centenarians in five areas around the world called the *Blue Zones*.[35]

There are various Harvard studies on longevity, including a twenty-six-year study of 160,000 American women who started the study at ages fifty to seventy-six. [36]

48

There is Jason Prall's film series titled *The Human Longevity Project,* about how he traveled the world looking at the healthiest people.[37]

There is Dr. Kelly Turner's study in her book titled *Radical Remission* on the common lifestyle factors that were present when certain people went into cancer remission statistically unexpectedly — her definition of "radical." These people used no conventional medicine; or, after trying conventional medicine with no results, they switched to alternative methods or used both.[38]

Distilling It Down: The Final Formula

The researchers all seem to be saying the same things. When it comes to health and longevity, the formula isn't that complicated.

Here is a compilation of the basics:

- Eat well. Eat more plants. Eat until only 80% full. Eat nutritiously. Change your diet. Limit alcohol.
- Move your body. Exercise. Be physically active. Detoxify your body through sweat. Control your weight.
- Lower stress. Cope effectively with stress. Know how to de-stress.
- Use herbs and supplements. Use plant-based remedies when possible.
- Be careful how you source your foods and products. Read labels.
- Get into natural sunlight. Get into nature.
- Get enough sleep.

- Release suppressed emotions. Increase positive emotions. Follow your intuition. Have a positive outlook. Be optimistic.
- Pray or meditate daily. Deepen your spiritual connection. Belong to a faith-based community.
- Embrace social support. Put family first. Spend time with friends and family. Create and nurture social circles. Love where you live and build community.
- Have a strong reason for living. Have a purpose.

Looking at it through the lens of The Self-Perpetuating Circle of Purpose:

BodyWork

- Eat well.
- Use herbs.
- Source products carefully.
- Exercise.
- Get into nature.
- Get enough sleep.

BrainWork

- Lower stress.
- Be optimistic.
- Follow your intuition.
- Pray or meditate daily.

WorldWork

- Belong to a faith-based community
- Put family and friends first.
- Have a purpose that energizes you.

The Sixty-Day Dare is created with these concepts in mind. It's a simple framework reflecting all three facets of these cultural behaviors within the broader facets of BodyWork, BrainWork, and WorldWork. We'll explore each in the coming chapters.

Looking for More Resources?

For more information and tips to complement what's already in the book and help you through your Sixty-Day Dare, download my *Reignite!* toolkit at AllisonMcCuneDavis.com/Toolkit. See the **download page at the back of the book for more details**.

Let the Four C's Lead Your Progress

It was funny, but when I was putting this book together, and I started looking at the behaviors needed to achieve the Sixty-Day Dare, I realized they all begin with C.

The Four Cs ask you to be:

- **Creative** in thinking outside the box and in being willing to have a paradigm shift.

- **Courageous** in breaking out of cycles of destructive habits and trying new things.
- **Committed** to dedicating yourself to that minimum of sixty days to create new habits.
- **Curious** to know yourself better, to ask questions, and to understand the world and why it has been hard to find the life you so deeply desire.

You will be amazed at what happens after doing something for sixty days in a row. Remember, our future is hidden in our daily routine.

PART TWO

BODYWORK

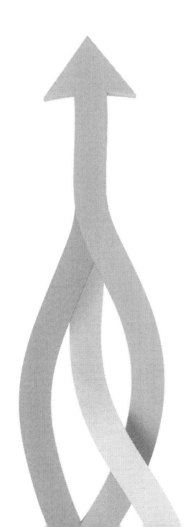

CHAPTER 4

The Body – Your Vessel for Life

Do not regret growing older. It's a privilege denied to many.
— MARK TWAIN

Your Healthy, Fit Body at 60

Approaching or turning sixty is, again, a big dang deal! Am I right, for goodness' sake? Yes, I am. You may only be fifty, or you may be beyond seventy. Everything here still holds true.

On my 60th birthday at the beach, I went to breakfast with my lifetime friend, who is a couple of years older than me. We sat at a darling outdoor table and drank delicious cappuccinos while leisurely enjoying our avocado toast. Our conversation was about social security and the pros and cons of taking it earlier or later. She had just recently figured this out.

I was interested, but I also thought, "Oh my goodness! Are we really talking about this?" It was one more reminder of the shock of entering my sixties.

These kinds of topics always lead my mind back to the crucial questions: Am I healthy enough? Am I doing everything right? What else should I do? Do you ever wonder about these things?

I'm guessing you might. I saw this funny, anonymous meme recently:

13-year-old me: "Don't tell me what to do!"

Me now: "Could someone tell me exactly, in chronological order and with great detail, what I have to do?"

Why Begin with the Body?

Why do we start with the physical aspect of health? Because it is almost always where everyone starts when they think about their health. In addition, if you are dealing with pain or something that physically limits you, this is the first thing on your mind. Therefore, improving the category of BodyWork can also significantly improve your BrainWork and WorldWork.

Before we go on, let's talk about what I mean by the term "BodyWork."

To many, bodywork means massage, chiropractic treatment, and the like — directly stimulating the physical body's muscles, bones, etc. I didn't realize how important bodywork was until my mid-40s to 50s. We live in a physical mass of muscles, bones, fascia, and lymph, and it needs to be moved, pressed on, rubbed, and dealt with. This type of bodywork can solve a multitude of problems.

However, in the Self-Perpetuating Circle of Purpose, this term means all the different work we do for and with our physical bodies.

To explore this facet, I'll tell you a little about my friend Gail.

Gail's Path to Health

It was around 2005, and we were at our usual weekly gathering of fellow homeschooling moms. Around five of us typically got together at the local children's art and science museum, letting our children run off energy and have fun with other kids while we moms got in some good adult time. Each of us had from two to five children ranging from nursing babies to about eight years old, so we had quite a crowd.

It was the beautiful beginning of our child-raising years when everything looked bright — but wow, were we busy and exhausted. We desperately needed our little group to keep our sanity.

That evening, we weren't in our normal meeting place. Instead, we had gathered at the home of a new member, Gail. As usual, we launched into one of our conversations about how to have better energy and a healthy family, eat good food, and avoid toxic products by reading labels.

Being new to the group, Gail had not yet talked to us in depth before. Mystified and a bit overwhelmed, she tried to follow the conversation. However, as she later told us, she was inwardly taken aback. "What are these women talking about?" she was thinking. "Probiotics? Grapefruit seed extract? Colloidal silver? I'm not even sure what those are. And I guess I need to start reading labels now?"

Over the weeks that followed, Gail started questioning everything she was doing. "What is actually in this toothpaste I'm using? Oh my gosh, my house is full of products with all kinds of toxins I can't pronounce! Where do I even begin fixing this?"

Slowly, Gail started learning about natural health. She began switching things out: Homemade laundry soap instead of detergent, healthy toothpaste instead of what the TV recommended, essential oil diffusers instead of scented candles or plug-in room deodorizers.

Gail was also having hormone difficulties. The toxins in those products are well known for being endocrine disrupters. She had very difficult menstrual cycles each month, where all she could do was lie on the couch for a day or two.

She didn't know why, but she gravitated to lavender oil. She began using it all the time — diffusing it in her home, inhaling it, and putting it topically on her body. The lavender, along with the change of home products, helped to normalize her cycles. Her endocrine system wasn't being disrupted anymore. That situation began a lifelong transformation for Gail.

The Rewards of Gail's Journey

Today, Gail is in her late fifties, married to a wonderful man, and her children are grown. She has six grandchildren she gets to help out with periodically. She and her husband are taking two years in their RV to travel around the United States, working various jobs. At the time of this writing, they are in Colorado working together for a company that has them walking outside in the gorgeous mountain air all day. They are getting paid to get healthy and see the world at the same time. They meet interesting new people, try out different churches in different locales, and love their lives.

Gail says she is much healthier now than she was twenty years ago. These days, she eats nutrient-dense food, gets enough water daily, takes her key supplements, herbs and oils, and exercises. Because of all of this, her sleep is good. She journals and reads a devotional every morning and is conscious of processing her emotions as they appear.

Gail believes that had she not become friends with natural, health-minded people, she probably would not be where she is today. It goes back to that concept of becoming like the five people we hang around.

Don't worry if you don't have friends who are working on their health in this way. There is a multitude online you can engage with, and honestly, there are probably people around you locally that you just haven't found yet. Many times, new people come to our natural health classes and say, "Oh my gosh, I didn't even know anything like this existed in our small town." We laugh and say, "Yes, we are the underground." Haha!

Let's take some wisdom from Gail's journey and look at the basics of what the body needs.

Natural Health in a Nutshell

One of the main tenets of holistic health is to eliminate the toxins and address the deficiencies in the body. You're either getting rid of something you don't need or adding something you do.

A foundational principle is that the human body is not deficient in anything synthetic. So why put synthetic substances like pharmaceuticals into it? They all have possible side effects.

The human body is not deficient in anything synthetic.

Supporting Health vs. Fighting Illness

Another foundational principle is understanding the difference between the germ theory and the terrain theory. Germ theory, typically followed by Western medicine, suggests that we should most concern ourselves with fighting off and killing bad germs and pathogens.

Terrain theory, more used by natural health practitioners, suggests we need to focus on a well-balanced, healthy body that will easily ward off pathogens, which are just a natural part of life, so we don't get sick.

Watching how your body reacts to various colds, flu, viruses, illnesses, etc., you can see how strong or weak it is and work on strengthening it.

In our world today, these fundamentals are rarely understood or employed. It's not our fault, but it is our problem. We are simply too far removed from living the much more natural life that existed only a few hundred years ago.

What The Human Body Needs to Support Health

Human bodies need some basic elements to maintain resilience and excellent health. This is a list of basics from my naturopath studies:

- Good Air
- Good Water
- Good Food
- Good Digestion
- Good Elimination – think "BULLS" (Bowels, Urinary, Lungs, Lymph, Skin)
- Good Hygiene – What goes on your skin goes into your bloodstream
- Good Exercise
- Good Sleep
- Emotional Balance
- Spiritual Balance

These fundamentals form the absolute foundation on which lasting health must be laid. Without that foundation, we will just get temporary relief from whatever we use, whether synthetic pills or natural herbs. However, if we have this key foundation in place, the body can do amazing things![39]

With this mentality, I've healed with natural solutions, treating periodontal disease (and avoiding its related surgery), a lifetime of environmental allergies, and UTI's, to name a few. In addition, our daughter from Ethiopia healed from giardia, a parasitic infection, through natural treatments.

Smart BodyWork Supports Health and Longevity

The longevity studies I mentioned earlier recommend eating well, using herbs and supplements, moving the body, and sleeping well as the primary keys to lasting health in the BodyWork department. This is no surprise to anyone, but it's nice to see the studies. Based on additional research, drinking pure water and breathing properly are also critical to good health.

Achieving Your Goals Requires Good Fitness

Think back to your goals after your self-evaluation. Where are you on your physical fitness journey? What are you physically able to do or not do at this point? How is that affecting your goals?

Now, think about the benefits of pursuing BodyWork and how it can help you get there. Here are just a few physical improvements you can have in your one-of-a-kind gift of a body:

- Better heart health – defying heart disease, the number one killer in America

- Better bone density and muscle mass – critically important at this age
- Reduced risk of chronic disease – typically environmentally caused
- Better lung function – we want strong lungs — it's all about oxygen
- Stronger immune system – so you don't get sick
- Better digestive/gut health – where 85 percent of our immune system resides
- Healthier skin and hair – of course! We want to look good!
- More physical energy – so you can do more without getting tired

In fact, all of these give us the ability to BE more active and live easily into old age.

It's part of that perpetuating circle. Do the foundational activities, get the benefits, and be able to do the foundational activities even better.

> *Do the foundational activities, get the benefits, and be able to do the foundational activities even better.*

If we do not do this, we will be miserable, sick, in bed, and depending on others for simple tasks. No one wants to live this way. If you already do, read on for some baby steps to move out of that.

And we haven't even talked about how these good things will uplift your mental state and how you operate in the world. That will come later.

Higher Energy Levels

When we pursue these BodyWork basics, our energy levels skyrocket. The more we do, the more energy we have.

How would you assess your energy levels? Do you have good energy for the day? Do you use lots of caffeine to prop you up? Do you just want to get back in bed more than you probably should?

Energy has been the key motivating word for me over the last twenty to thirty years as I've raised my children. I think it is for everyone.

Today, my energy levels are solid, but twenty years ago, I realized I was getting the flu about every six weeks and would be in bed for an entire week. This totally impacted my ability to be a good mom (or at least feel like I was). Finally, I found my first naturopath doctor in Oklahoma. He did all kinds of testing. Sex hormones, neuro hormones, blood, poop, urine, hair follicle for heavy metals, etc.

We realized my adrenals were "shot" (his word). I had too much harmful and not enough beneficial bacteria in my gut, and my thyroid wasn't working well either. We started addressing these issues with herbs, vitamins, minerals, and diet, including raw milk. It took a while, but eventually, my attention to these paid off.

I eat much better now, but again, our food is missing so many minerals from being grown in soil that it just doesn't compare to food from the old days. So, I absolutely take my vitamins and minerals. They are key for my energy levels, though it took me a long time to get into a good habit. I used to forget to take them all the time. That's why this book includes some great tips for remembering to do your new habits.

The other main key to my energy increase was exercise. There is just no denying what seems to be a paradox, but it is how the body works. The more energy we spend exercising, the more energy we get back. It's supply and demand (up to a point). Kinda like nursing a baby. The more you nurse (slowly increasing), the more milk your body creates (as long as you drink lots of water and eat good food). The more you exercise (slowing increasing as you are able), the more energy your body creates. What a beautiful thing our bodies are!

When, at 55, I finally decided to start exercising regularly, I believed I could only commit to twice a week. I worked at that for two years, increasing to three times a week midway through. When we went on family hikes around that same time, I noticed I was breathing more easily and didn't have to stop as often. That was extremely motivating.

Over the following two years, I increased to four and then five times a week. That was how I could finish 75 Hard, which included those two 45-minute exercise sessions daily, one outside in the elements.

It was absolutely not too late for me, nor is it for you. If all you can do is walk to the stop sign and back, then that is where you start. It's all good!

Don't forget about Joan MacDonald on Instagram. Remember? The 78-year-old that started at 70!

Better Mobility

What fun is living a long life if you can't get around?

The CDC shows that the stats could be better in the United States for the recommended physical activity of at least 150 minutes a week of moderate-intensity exercise or 75 minutes a week of vigorous exercise plus at least two days a week of strength training. 17.6 percent of women ages 50–64 are doing this. Only 10.8 percent of women over 65 are doing this.[40]

If we want good mobility, again, we must use our bodies. Don't let that amount of exercise time overwhelm you, though. Remember. Baby steps.

While my mother was alive during her last few years, her late seventies to early eighties, she had very limited mobility and serious mental decline. I hated seeing it. Her inattention to these basics finally caught up with her.

And I get it. Before the decline started, she was just living her happy life. Four children and thirteen grandchildren who all adored her. All her dogs and cats. Good friends. She was happy. She wasn't thinking about exercising.

Then, the decline started.

The muscles in her legs deteriorated. At first, she needed a cane. Then, she moved into a wheelchair. She wasn't eating enough protein and probably ate too much sugar. I have to fight that same tendency myself. She likely needed more supplements and definitely a fitness routine earlier on. She did enjoy playing golf in her younger years but had left that behind.

It's hard when loved ones get older. We all do our best to make their last years good, but many times, it is too little too late. Thank goodness my middle sister, Evie, could take care of her during that last year.

You are just like a car. You need the right fuel and the right oil and maintenance to last a long time. "Use it, or lose it," plus good fuel, is the mantra for mobility.

You are just like a car. You need the right fuel and the right oil and maintenance to last a long time.

At my current age, when I get up from sitting for too long, my joints definitely talk to me. However, if it's a day when I'm moving a lot — walking, running errands, moving through the house, or whatever — I never notice that.

Taking some key supplements helps, too. I have experimented with discontinuing them. After about 7-10 days, I start feeling achy joints again, even while moving, mostly in my hands, feet, and knees. For many, supplements are an easy fix and definitely something to try. Talk to your wellness practitioner to get recommendations. Definitely start here first rather than a prescription medication. Why add the side effects of a prescription if you don't have to?

Go Back to the Garden of Eden

In many of my classes, I've used this scenario: Imagine you live outdoors in the Garden of Eden. You walk through it day and night, barefoot on top of leaves and plants that are on your path. You smell all the trees and flowers and plants each day. All day. You brush by bushes, and the limbs and leaves invisibly push their fragrance into the air and into your nose. This is your norm. Your body is getting what it needs by living in this place. Fresh air, plant life, movement, good soil for your food, good water, and the sun.

When we don't live this way, instead caging ourselves in our modern houses with electricity and all the conveniences too numerous to list, our bodies begin to crave certain foods and smells. It's important to acknowledge these.

It's fascinating to see which plant smells you are attracted to or turned off by. It gives us clues as to what is going on with your body and what areas need attention.

Let's look at a simple way that simple things can absolutely move us in the right direction: That lavender oil Gail was so attracted to went directly into her nose as she inhaled, passed the blood-brain barrier, and moved into the limbic system of her brain. There, it stirred the places where memory, trauma, and emotion reside. When applied topically, it seeped into her skin and then her bloodstream. Those small molecules traveled to the correct cells in her body and began to bring things into homeostasis. Her body began to heal. This is just one way, a very pleasant way, we can help our bodies heal. (Always use the highest-grade oils.)

Self-Reflection: Where Are You with BodyWork?

How does your body feel right now? Do you feel like you have the energy to do the things you want to do, or do you constantly struggle? Have you been checked recently for bone density? What's your muscle mass? Do you always get sick, or is your immune system well-tuned? Do you eat too much sugar or foods that quickly turn to sugar, like wheat?

If you could change something, what would it be? Keep that in mind as we start into the next chapter, where you'll decide what you want to work on in the BodyWork part of the Sixty-Day Dare.

You are on the way to making big changes in your life through small, incremental steps. Keep your mind focused not just on the question "Where do I want to be in five or ten years?" but also, "How do I want to feel in sixty days?"

With that in mind, let's start looking at the Big Five BodyWork options.

CHAPTER 5

The BodyWork Big Five

Those who have no time for healthy eating will
sooner or later have to find the time for illness.
— EDWARD STANLEY

Based on research into longevity, I have created five simple options for BodyWork (and for each of the other two categories). The Big Five take all that research into account to give the best benefits.

Remember: **You only have to pick one** of the options below for your Sixty-Day Dare. This is what you will choose to do every day for sixty days. Having options gives you some flexibility to suit your own needs.

The BodyWork Big Five are:

- **EAT** – Pick one thing you will add, subtract, or change about what or how you are eating to improve your health.
- **DRINK** – Drink at least half your body weight in ounces of water.
- **MOVE** – Exercise for a set number of minutes per day, ideally 45 minutes, but if you need to do less, that is completely fine. You decide where you will start. You can even start at a lower amount and aim to reach a higher one by the end of your 60 days.
- **SLEEP** – Get at least seven hours of true sleep each night. Eight or nine would be wonderful.
- **BREATHE** – Do at least 10 minutes of deep breathing a day.

Almost all wellness practitioners would agree that these five fundamentals are key. Get these going in the right direction, and you will be miles ahead on your wellness path.

Remember, we're taking baby steps. Even doing one of these will get you on a much better track. To help you choose, let's look at some guidelines and ideas for each option.

#1: EAT – Guidelines and Ideas

This option is very flexible. The goal is to do something related to eating a healthier diet, but you get to pick what works for you. You could get advice from your doctor or, better yet, someone skilled in nutrition. I'm not going to dictate a diet to you.

Ideas

Here are some ideas for choosing this option (remember, you just have to do one of these, not ALL of them!):

- Go on a clean diet — eliminate all toxins, chemicals, and processed foods. Focus on getting good protein and veggies.
- Go on a specific, health-focused diet such as food combining or intermittent fasting. Get a good book like *Good Energy* or *The Fast Metabolism Diet*[41] (good books to learn the basics of good eating).
- Get an app or tracking device such as the Lumen and track your macros (fats, protein, and carbs) to control how many you get each day. You can also get a continuous glucose monitoring device (CGM) that tracks how your food affects your glucose. This is highly motivating. Check out Levels.com.
- Add something beneficial to your diet, like a certain number of servings of vegetables and/or fruits daily or a certain number of grams of protein daily.
- Eliminate certain potentially inflammatory or otherwise harmful items like wheat, dairy, or alcohol.
- Decide to start on a set of vitamins and/or supplements every day to help your health. (Talk to your health practitioner about your specific situation, as these sometimes may interfere with certain medications, etc.)

A Note on Alcohol

"A little red wine" was listed as something those in the Blue Zones did (except in Loma Linda, CA). Probably because they were so healthy in every other way, their bodies could metabolize it easily. However, more research has shown that alcohol is a toxin and prevents many necessary bodily processes from happening, including getting a good night's sleep. Talk to your health practitioner if you have questions about alcohol and your own situation.

Start Smart: Know What You're Eating

Studying the explorers listed in Chapter Two reveals an emphasis on nutrient-dense foods with some meat and lots of plants. When we eat meat, we want grass-fed and grass-finished beef if possible. We want free-range, organic eggs and chicken. We want wild-caught salmon and fish. Probably not pork, and probably not bottom-dwelling fish like catfish. These are scavenger animals eating nasty things that are better left to them.

Critical Point: Women our age need to build and keep muscle, which is vital for our health. To gain muscle, we need protein. Eat good beef, salmon, chicken, and eggs weekly. If you're a vegetarian, you'll need to take extra care to make sure you get enough protein.

If you consume dairy, you want raw milk, cream, and cheese, not homogenized and pasteurized. Raw dairy is very healing to the body and, in the old days, was used by doctors to cure all sorts of gut issues.[42] [43] You'll find these dairy items at local family farms. You also want organic fruits and vegetables. Search online for the Dirty Dozen list to see which are most important to be organic.

If you are concerned about the cost, remember that your money will be better spent on smarter eating than on sick care down the road. I know many people who have lots of kids and are on very tight budgets, and they organize their spending wisely to eat their best. Even if you have insurance, healthcare is costly, especially when you have chronic issues.

> *Your money will be better spent on smarter eating than on sick care down the road*

Supplements Count

Yes, you can choose to add supplements under the EAT category if you pick it as your BodyWork option.

I've been taking supplements for over thirty years, and if I stop (which I have done, just to see what happens), I don't feel as good. My joints hurt. My hormone tests and blood tests come back with worse results. My energy level is low.

Most wellness professionals advise taking some basic vitamins like D and K2, B complex, magnesium, omega 3s, probiotics, a multivitamin, and zinc. I add others for joint function, collagen production, sleep help, and more. There is much more to the world of supplements, and every natural health practitioner or functional medical doctor sells the ones they prefer.

One supplement I really love is wolfberry, which I mentioned before. When researching the centenarians in Ningxia, China, Dr. Young came to believe that this food, which is massively high in antioxidants, was a major contributing factor to their long lives. Ten years before Young's journey, an interesting study was done:

> According to a report from the State Scientific and Technological Commission of China, the wolfberry fruits were effective in increasing white blood cells, protecting the liver, relieving hypertension, and displaying an insulin-like action that was effective in promoting fat decomposition and reducing blood sugar. The commission also noted that a wolfberry extract inhibited cancer growth by 58 percent.[44]

It also has eyesight benefits, and I attribute my really good eyesight at sixty-three to wolfberry.

#2: DRINK — Guidelines and Ideas

Think of water as the gas in your car, but also like the oil. It lubricates everything. Our internal organs need to be saturated with water.

Our bodies are made up of 60 percent water. The lungs are 80 percent water, the muscles are 75 percent water, the brain is 81 percent water, the skin is 64 percent water, the blood is 91 percent water, the cartilage is 55 percent water, and the bones are 13 percent. That's a lot of water!

Think about our veins and arteries. Do we want them hard and brittle or supple and pliable? That visual really helped me desire more water. It's vital to every cell. Ample water fights viral attacks. It cleanses the kidneys. The liver requires water above all substances to function. Water flushes out waste and toxins. It lubricates tissues and joints, regulates temperature, moisturizes the skin, and creates equilibrium.[45]

If your goal is to lose weight, drinking enough water is one key to that process. I've seen the weight go or stay according to whether I'm drinking enough water.

How Much?

For The Sixty-Day Dare, **if you choose water, you'll need to drink at least half your body weight in ounces each day.** That is the general guideline from multiple sources.

This may feel like a lot, but it's not. Drinking too much water is possible, but it's rare. It typically only happens with extreme athletes.

However, if you have kidney or heart disease, or if you want to drink more than half your body weight in ounces, talk to your doc about how much water you should drink.

What Kind?

This is a big controversy. In my naturopath studies, we had an entire section on water. Ideally, water should be from natural springs. Second-best is a reverse-osmosis (RO) system for your kitchen sink. A plumber can install this.

I drink both and keep bottled spring water on hand for those times when I am moving fast and just need to grab a bottle on the go, but mostly, I love using my stainless steel cups. Plastic is not good for our bodies.

If you don't want to spend the money to get an RO system, at least purchase some sort of water filter. It is definitely better than nothing.

#3: MOVE – Guidelines and Ideas

If you can't fly, run. If you can't run, walk.
If you can't walk, crawl, but by all means, keep moving.
— MARTIN LUTHER KING, JR.

Exercise Ideas

Here are some exercise suggestions (you can mix these together or not as you like; just make sure to get in your set amount of time each day):

- **Strength Training:** Pilates, weightlifting (starting with small weights still has benefits!)
- **Low-intensity cardio:** Walking, low-impact aerobics
- **Flexibility:** Yoga, stretching

Tips for Success

I listen to all kinds of experts on the subject of health and muscles. Most say that for women over 50, muscle strength is the number one consideration. We must build muscle to stay mobile and strong as we enter these next decades. Strength training is, therefore, crucial. If you've picked "Move" for your BodyWork option, I'd advise incorporating strength training at least a couple of times each week.

For instance, I do a 40-minute Pilates reformer class three days a week and a weightlifting session two days a week for strength. My low-intensity cardio is walking as often as possible, whether outside or on the treadmill, usually for 30-60 minutes at a time. You obviously don't have to do all of that if you're just starting out. It's just an example of how you could combine things.

This Pub Med Study shows us that walking is a beneficial, easy, low-intensity exercise. The world's largest research project, comprised of 17 studies and 227,000 people around the world, shows that the more you walk, the lower your risk of death, even if you walk the minimum recommendation of four thousand steps. And the more steps, the better.[46]

For flexibility, just get a yoga mat, sit down on the floor, and stretch your body. Find some YouTube videos to follow along with. Even 10 minutes is good. If you do more than this, go you!!

Feeling Down or Anxious? Exercise Could Help

Exercise is an antidote to depression and anxiety.[47] More oxygen into the body is always a good thing. If you deal with these issues, maybe MOVE is the BodyWork choice for you. Get outside and MOVE that body! It will absolutely help.

For years, I have followed business and fitness expert Chalene Johnson online and gone to many of her conferences. One of my favorite quotes from her is, "People ask me how often they should exercise, and I ask them, 'Well, how often do you want to be in a good mood?'"

It is exercise alone that supports the spirits
and keeps the mind in vigor.
— MARCUS TULLIUS CICERO

#4: SLEEP – Guidelines and Ideas

Seventy million Americans do not get enough sleep. Historically, 100 years ago, we slept nine hours a night. Many say the invention of the light bulb is where more disease started by messing up our healthy circadian rhythm — getting up with the sun and going to bed when it got dark outside.

Even if your diet is good, if your sleep is off, your health can go awry. Getting enough good sleep is critical for so many aspects of our health: repairing and healing, regulating mood, brain function, chronic illness, diabetes, heart disease, cancer, and Alzheimer's. If you struggle with sleep and have issues such as those in this list, focusing on this area could help. It might be the perfect BodyWork option for you.

Even more important, you may not even know how it's affecting you.

Business and fitness expert Chalene Johnson has a story I like to share.[48] In her early fifties, she visited Dr. Daniel Amen, a psychiatrist and brain disorder specialist who developed a mode of scanning and getting 3D pictures of the brain. She was sure her scans would reveal that she was one of the healthiest people they had ever seen.

The doctor entered the room with scans in hand, sat down, and said, "Well, either you are a heroin addict, or you have been a prisoner of war."

Stunned, she said, "What in the world are you talking about?"

"You have various areas on your brain that are consistent with those groups of people. Drugs or sleep deprivation is the cause. This will lead to dementia in not too many years. How much do you sleep?

"Uh oh. I've been sleeping four to five hours a night for years." She is just one of those fast-moving people who didn't think she needed that much sleep. She was wrong.

The good news is that the body heals. She could heal her brain with various supplements and good sleep methods. Since then, she has prioritized her sleep and gets at least seven hours or more a night.

Why Can't We Sleep?

Dr. Mark Hyman tells us there are many potential root causes of sleep problems.

- A diet high in starch and carbohydrates, which causes blood-sugar fluctuations.
- Alcohol and/or caffeine consumption.
- Going to bed tired and wired without discharging chronic stress first. This practice creates adrenal issues and causes the body to produce too much cortisol, the fight-or-flight hormone.
- A lack of magnesium causes irritability, tension, and stress.
- Lack of muscle or strength training.
- Getting up to pee multiple times a night. This interferes with sleep and can also be a symptom of another issue that needs to be checked out.
- Health issues such as undiagnosed sleep apnea, a deviated septum, thyroid issues, inflammation in the body or brain, or hormonal imbalances.[49]

Start Smart with Sleep

If you've chosen Sleep as your BodyWork option, investing in a sleep tracker at the beginning can be very useful. For instance, the Oura Ring allows you to see how much deep sleep, REM sleep, and light sleep you get each night. Also, you can see the levels of stress you have all day long and whether you have gotten enough restorative time during the day.

At the minimum, you'll need to set a goal to get to bed — preferably at the same time each night. You can also do many other things to help you sleep, from making sure you see sunlight several hours a day to a completely dark bedroom at night.

#5: BREATHE – Guidelines and Ideas

It's not like we can accidentally not breathe. Are we really going to count breathing in the Big Five?

Yes, we are. Trust me. First, let's look at the benefits of doing breathwork, which are too important to dismiss.

The Benefits of Better Breathing

Information on the breath has been around for thousands of years in the world of monasteries and yoga but is only recently going mainstream. Since we Americans need our scientific studies, here's some data for you.

Wim Hof, a 65-year-old Dutch extreme athlete, was studied for his ability to control his endocrine and immune systems. He recommends a deep-breathing method that alters the body chemistry, causing temporary alkalosis (high alkalinity of the blood and body fluids) and activating the good stress response, forcing the body to adapt, strengthen, and build resistance.

The results are complex to explain, but basically, what happens is that this breathing increases the concentration of red blood cells. The oxygen held in red blood cells floods into the tissues. Lung capacity and circulation improve, and your metabolism becomes more efficient.

Through this deep breathing, Hof has shown he is able to control various functions of his body. He says anyone can do this and also heal from a variety of chronic illnesses. Auto-immune, Crohn's disease, arthritis, and more.

The autonomic nervous system is supposed to be beyond our control — the heart, various organs, the immune system — but, through scientific testing, Hof showed the ability to radically influence those functions through breathing and mental focus. For these exercises, Hof says to breathe through either your nose or mouth, whichever helps you get the deepest breaths.[50]

Gary Brecka, a human biologist, tells us to "get addicted to breath work. It's one of the most important practices we can do daily, and it's free! It will improve your emotional state, longevity, and digestion of nutrients. It will also help you handle anxiety and depression and will help the bio-bacteria in the gut perform better."[51]

He recommends the Wim Hof process too. Gary says this can be so beneficial to someone with asthma, anxiety, high blood pressure, and more. I love his line, "The presence of oxygen is the absence of disease."[52] Let's get to breathing correctly!

Breathing: Are You Doing It Wrong?

Journalist James Nestor studied every facet of the breath and recently wrote an award-winning book, *Breath*, on the subject. He says that, based on his research, you might be doing everything else right — food, exercise, sleep — but if you are not breathing correctly, you will still have problems.[53]

Yes, believe it or not, you can breathe incorrectly.

I learned much about breathing when I started yoga a quarter century ago and eventually got certified. One thing I learned is that Americans don't breathe correctly:

- We breathe too much, too shallowly, in the upper part of our chests. This causes us to offload too much carbon dioxide and not absorb enough oxygen.
- We inhale through our mouths, which creates additional problems by not filtering the air through our noses. Nose breathing slows down the incoming air and filters, humidifies, and conditions it so the lungs can absorb the oxygen much more easily. The nose also produces nitric oxide, a molecule that is a vaso-dilator (dilates blood vessels, which decreases blood pressure). Nitric oxide plays an essential role in oxygen delivery and fights off pathogens — it's

our first line of defense against illness. Due to its dilation of the blood vessels, we get 20 percent more oxygen breathing through the nose than through the mouth.[54]

Be Mindful to Breathe Well

To breathe correctly, we first have to be aware of how we're breathing. The #1 mantra in yoga is "It is all about the breath." When we move through yoga poses, we always focus on the breath while trying to get our bodies in the pose correctly. This process forces us to focus our minds. You don't have to do yoga to follow this guideline. Throughout the day, take a moment to check how you're breathing and make adjustments where needed.

Ideas for doing BREATHE as your BodyWork

It might seem funny to think about purposely doing something you already do without thinking, but it's not quite as easy as just continuing to breathe. Doing mindful breathwork is different. Here are some ideas for incorporating it as your BodyWork option:

- Use a specific breathwork technique, such as the Wim Hof method (more on that in this section).
- Get a breathwork app and do the exercises with it each day.
- Incorporate essential oils into your breathwork sessions.

Breathwork Techniques

There are many different kinds of breathwork. Here are some basics to try:

- Breathe in for five to six seconds and out for five to six seconds. You can focus on that kind of slow breathing through the nose throughout the day.[55]
- Take thirty or so deep breaths in and out; after the last exhale, hold your breath as long as possible, then take a deep breath and hold it for 15 seconds, then start over. Three to four rounds is a good practice.[56]
- Use essential oils to enhance your breathwork. High-grade oils contain molecules so small that when inhaled (and also when used topically or ingested), they travel to the cellular level in just a few minutes. When inhaled into the limbic system, the seat of emotions and trauma, certain essential oils can bring much healing. In addition, oils like peppermint or eucalyptus can help clear the lungs and/or sinuses to get that deep breath if you're struggling with a cold or flu. They also help get rid of headaches. Rub the oil in your hands, cup your hands up to your nose and mouth, and take deep breaths.

Caution! Source Your Supplies Carefully

When purchasing anything you plan to put in, on, or around your body, remember: High grade is crucial.

Many supplements and other alternative treatments, such as essential oils, are not regulated in the United States. Do your research and get them from a trusted source — direct from a reputable seller is best. Do not buy them from online marketplaces or big-box retailers, as the quality isn't guaranteed. There are many cases of shady sellers in online marketplaces pushing fake knockoffs with labels that look like they come from a reputable seller. And the brands through big-box retailers are often sub-par quality. My *Reignite!* toolkit includes some recommendations. Most reputable naturopaths, chiropractors, or holistic medicine specialists will have good advice, too.

Which Should I Choose?

You've already done some self-evaluations earlier in the book. Were any in the BodyWork areas low numbers? That will definitely give you a hint for a starting place. Pick the one looming largest in your mind.

If you are at the beginning of this new mindset, you might think you need work in every category and want to do them all. However, there's a reason why I want you to pick just one. Trying to do several things at once can get overwhelming, which might cause you to burn out. Keep it simple. Remember, this is a START.

If you are already doing well in all areas of the BodyWork Big Five, then you could pick something that increases the benefit of what you're already doing.

For instance, if you are already walking 30 minutes a day before you start the Sixty-Day Dare, you could still choose "MOVE" but add some 15-minute weightlifting sessions each day to equal the 45 minutes, with lower-body weights three days a week and upper-body the other three days a week, and a stretching session on the seventh day. This would expand your existing habit to include all three important areas of MOVE: Walking, lifting weights, and stretching.

Or maybe you have a fairly good diet but are concerned with the level of sugar or alcohol you consume, so you decide to limit or eliminate those two things for your Sixty-Day Dare.

Speaking of simple, if you're just starting down this road and you're looking for the simplest options with the most benefits, pick either exercise or water. When it comes to doing something for sixty days, this will be the best and easiest place to start, AND it will make a big difference.

Change Your Mindset and the Rest Will Follow

So, have you decided on an option you'll commit to for sixty days?

If you're having trouble deciding, don't worry — the next chapter can help.

For now, let's get that beautiful mind of yours thinking, "I can do this." Remember, you will design this plan with your success in mind.

Think back to my experience of 75 Hard. The day I heard about it, I thought there was no way in hell I could ever do it. Four months later, I decided I could. And then, I did. That was all due to a mindset shift. Nothing else.

I know you've got the ability to make a mindset shift, too.

How can you make it doable yet challenging enough to push you? Remember: baby steps. We are going to baby-step our way to really good habits. It goes back to that oh-so-true line: "Our future is hidden in our daily routine."

Once you've picked your option, write it down. Don't worry; it's not set in stone until your official start date. In the next chapter, you'll find some creative tips for making this fun — and maybe even easier than you might think. Once you read on and start planning, the seemingly impossible option you didn't choose might suddenly look a lot more possible.

CHAPTER 6

Planning Your BodyWork

Setting goals is the first step in turning the invisible into the visible.
— TONY ROBBINS

Smart Choices Should Be Fun and Achievable

Now that you've made your BodyWork choice, let's talk about how to make it work for you. The goal is to make your next sixty days as pleasant and enjoyable as possible yet also a bit of a challenge. I predict this process will make you excited about your future. Things are definitely looking up, my dear! You've got this!

SMART Goals Create Clarity

As you begin to plan, one of the first things you may have noticed is that the BodyWork options are designed in the framework of SMART Goals. I'm sure many of you know about this principle, but if not, I will outline it here.

SMART is an acronym for:

Specific
Measurable
Achievable
Relevant
Time-Based

All your goals should be SMART. I've created the Big Five options using this SMART framework so that you will be very clear about whether you are achieving them.

Let's look at an example.

This is how you would make the MOVE choice a SMART goal for The Sixty-Day Dare.

Make it **Specific**: I will exercise for X minutes every day for 60 days in a row.

Make it **Measurable**. "30 minutes, every day for 60 days" is easy to measure.

Hopefully, you feel this goal is **Achievable**. If not, you will feel too demotivated to try. (If you do realize your initial goal is not realistic for your starting point, there's an adjustment allowance, too, which I'll get to shortly.)

It is **Relevant** if you know you need to do it.

It is clearly **Time-based**. You have said how long you will walk, that you will walk every day, and that this will go on for 60 days.

Need to Adjust? That's Okay

If you feel the recommended goal is not achievable, you can adjust it to fit your situation. For instance, maybe you haven't exercised in years, and you're not sure how long you can walk. It's all right to lessen the time you commit to walking each day. There is nothing wrong with saying you will walk at least 20 minutes each day. If you feel like going further on certain days, great! And even if you don't, you still achieve the goal.

You can also adjust to a realistically challenging baseline after you begin — but only once. So, within your first week, if you realize you set a goal that's just not realistic, you can adjust it accordingly. However, after that, you're committed. So, adjust wisely!

One great way to start small and continually challenge yourself is to create a goal in the SMART framework to increase over time. So, your goal could be to start with only five minutes of exercise on the first day and do one more minute each day till you get to 45, after which you do that for the rest of the 60 days. All of that is still in the SMART framework.

A Few More SMART Tips

As you set your goals, ask yourself whether you're being specific enough to measure.

If you've chosen EAT, and you're going to go on a certain food plan, then your measurement is whether you stuck to that plan for that day. If you deviated even slightly, you didn't stick to the plan. If you're deciding on what to eliminate or add to your diet, you'd need to specify exactly what those are. For instance, instead of, "Every day, I'll take magnesium and vitamin D," it would be better to say, "Every day, I'll take 300 mg of magnesium and 4000 IU of vitamin D, once per day."

When you use these parameters, you clearly know whether you achieved the goal or not.

Shoot for the moon. Even if you miss,
you'll land among the stars.
— **LES BROWN**

Be Curious: You Are Now a Health Detective

For a dozen years, I have used this phrase, "Be your own health detective."

To really change our lives, we must go beyond just taking some superficial actions and dive deep into how our bodies work.

Certainly, the BodyWork Big Five will help you in a multitude of ways, no matter what is going on. However, you might also want to dig a little deeper into the root causes of any ailments. As we saw when looking into the Self-Perpetuating Circle of Purpose, everything is connected.

For instance, you may think SLEEP is your best BodyWork Big Five option. However, if the reason you're not sleeping is due to a lack of nutrients, then you might be better off addressing the nutrient issue by choosing EAT. This choice would probably help many other things while also helping you sleep.

There are many, many ways to educate yourself. Join some natural health women's groups on social media. There are soooooo many, and some with thousands of people. Ask those people for ways to find more answers. Find an in-person group in your local area. Look for books by knowledgeable authors. Listen to podcasts. Most of all, ask questions. The more you know, the better you'll be able to address your situation.

If you're unsure how to assess reputable sources, make an appointment with a natural health practitioner to get some guidance on your journey. You might already have a medical doctor that you can get a diagnosis from if you don't know what is going on. That can be a good start. Then, let your doctor know you plan on adding some new healthy lifestyle practices. I'm guessing they will be happy about that and encourage you.

The key is to take an interest and try to learn something new — whether it's from your doctor or from research. Whatever you find out about your health, make sure you investigate all the options available to you.

Auto-Immune Disorders as An Example

President and CEO of Autoimmune Association, Molly Murray, states that "auto-immune diseases affect 50 million Americans. However, given the complexity... this is likely an underestimate. Even more alarming, autoimmunity is reaching epidemic levels, with some studies estimating an increase of 3–12 percent annually."[57]

I was just talking to Carol, who, at 57, was recently diagnosed with a rare kind of auto-immune disorder. She felt she had no choice but to get on medication just to be able to function, but once she felt better, she started her research and began making lifestyle changes. Lab reports showed she could, little by little, get off all of her medications. She says she has to be very conscious not to trigger a flare-up. The two main components to protect against that are good sleep and controlling her stress. So, for someone like her, those might be key areas to pursue in a Sixty-Day Dare.

Dealing with Side Effects

The problem with medications is they have side effects that can confuse the issues, making it hard to figure out if your original problem is getting better. When someone is taking multiple prescription medications, I think, "Oh my goodness. How do you even know what is going on? What is causing what?"

The best approach is to take one issue at a time and try to solve it naturally, hopefully weaning off medication. If you feel this is something you want to attempt, research the side effects your medications could be causing. With your doctor's supervision, start weaning off the medication that is least concerning to stop taking. You'll want to also ensure you are addressing the root cause the medication was meant to address.

Be Creative: Find Ways to Make It Fun and Easy

When making major changes, the little things can make a big difference in sticking to them or not.

James Clear, author of *Atomic Habits*, gives us these four guidelines for building better habits. "Make it obvious... Make it attractive...Make it easy...Make it satisfying."[58]

You will have to decide what is in your budget, but here are just a few ways I have found to make things more enjoyable in the BodyWork department. I'm sure there are many others.

Redesign Your Eating Environment

Redesign your kitchen to place the healthy food items in your direct eyesight first. Remember this: Environment triggers behavior!

Fresh fruit and veggies in clear glass bowls at eye level in the fridge make a big difference.

Get rid of the unhealthy food so you are not tempted. If you want a food item that you've limited, require yourself to go out of your house to get it. Many times, that makes it easy not to eat it. If others in your house eat a food you're tempted by that isn't on your plan, let them know you'll place it in a certain closed cabinet or somewhere in the fridge where you won't see it as easily.

Make Drinking Fun

Find some cute water bottles and dedicate them to your water intake. I like having two stainless steel 32-ounce cups. I fill them up at bedtime or in the morning for the day. I keep one with me at home throughout the day and set the other on my entry table to make it easy to grab when I'm going out.

Get Enthused about Exercise

Lay your exercise clothes and your shoes out at night so they are the first things you see when you wake up. Then, don't think about it — just put them on!

One of the best thoughts that helped me as I started exercising regularly was this: Just lace up your shoes. Don't think about anything but that. Once they are on, you will be much more ready to walk out the door and go for that walk, head to the gym, or do whatever other exercise you've planned.

Just lace up your shoes.

After I started exercising regularly, I purchased some cute exercise clothes. This helped. You want to enjoy putting those clothes on and looking like an exercise diva! Of course, you need good walking shoes if you will be walking. And good socks too!

For my exercise outfit, the bottom is leggings — full length for winter, ¾ length for fall and spring and sometimes summer, and 10" legging shorts for summer. Those go to right above my knee. That's as short as I'm going! On top, I like a fun short-sleeved T-shirt or cute sleeveless workout shirts for the summer that are long enough to cover my butt. That's me. You do you!

Sleep Better and Love It

If you will be working on your sleep during this time, let's go back to thinking about your environment.

Make your bedroom a sanctuary. Make it calm, serene, beautiful. A place you love to enter. Remove anything in there that signifies activity. Replace lamp bulbs with amber, blue-blocking light bulbs. Blue light wakes you up; you don't want that when you're trying to sleep. Wear blue-blocking glasses in the hour or two before bedtime.

Honestly, any children's pictures should go somewhere else in the house. If you have a partner, those kids' photos just ain't good to have in the bedroom for all the love going on between you two, if you know what I mean. The pictures can go in any other room in the house. In the bedroom, put up soothing artwork, such as landscapes. You can find things at thrift stores that will fit just about any budget.

Breathe Deeply

For breathwork, the most enjoyable app I have found is the Wim Hof app. (I mentioned Wim Hof in the Breathwork section of the last chapter.) There is a monthly fee, but you could try it for a month and see if you like it. It keeps track of your breathwork plus other activities, guides you through each session, allows you to set different variables, and includes badges to earn. It's funny how those can be motivating.

In addition, if you need help remembering to do it, maybe set up a little frame on your bedside with a reminder note to yourself in it or put a reminder on your phone that comes up at a specific time.

Your timing can also be creative. Doing breathwork in bed before I get up is my solution for remembering to do it. Once the day gets going, it is easier to forget. Also, the timing is perfect because breathwork connects and activates the hormonal, immune, and nervous systems — a great way to start the day.

As I mentioned before, combining essential oils is another way to enhance breathwork. If you want to add essential oils to your routine or improve your habit of engaging in a breathing session with them, put them somewhere you will see them when you need them. I have mine on my coffee table in the room where I sit and drink my coffee in the morning and think about my day. They are sitting on a beautiful little silver tray. Remember: Make it attractive!

Be Courageous: Challenge Yourself

Of the three sections, BodyWork, BrainWork, and WorldWork, I think the BodyWork section can be the most challenging, depending on what you choose and your current lifestyle. That might not be true for everyone, of course. We are all different.

Part of the reason it feels challenging is that it pushes you to go where you're not comfortable. The only way to do something new is to rev up that courage that is, no doubt, inside you and move out of your comfort zone. Little by little. Step by step.

Remember: This is just a simple mindset change.

The reason people don't achieve their dreams is that they aren't willing to move out of that comfy little spot they love to lounge in. Hey, it's ok to be there sometimes. Look at getting to be in your comfy place as a reward for making those efforts.

For instance, I would love to sit and needlepoint all day. It's one of my favorite hobbies, and it's a cozy activity.

However, I don't let myself do it until I have achieved certain things during the day. I like to reward myself with this hobby because it produces a beautiful heirloom that I can pass down to my children someday.

While I needlepoint, I always listen to an audiobook or podcast or watch a TV show. Find a reward you love and feel good about engaging in — but only after you've done your Sixty-Day Dare activities and any other important tasks for the day.

Be Committed: Design a Foolproof BodyWork System

Let's start by looking at your calendar and deciding your Start Day — the day your Sixty-Day Dare will commence. What's a good day for that?

This is not necessarily just picking a day. If you have any travel days in the sixty-day period, you will need to decide if you can still accomplish your goal during that time and plan to make that happen. Travel doesn't need to present a problem, but you do need to think it through.

Ask yourself questions. "If I'm traveling, and MOVE is my option, can I get some walking in during that day somehow? When exactly will I do that? If EAT is my choice, what will my food choices be? Do I need to bring something with me? Are restaurants available that will have what I need to eat to stay on my Sixty-Day Dare?"

Sit down and make some notes about what you need to purchase or how you need to rearrange your days. Do you need to opt out of any of your normal activities to give yourself time to accomplish your goals? Do you need to say no to anyone? Strong boundaries will be essential to your success with these sixty days. We will talk more about boundaries later, but for now, know you need them!

Talk to your family and let them know you are doing this, and you could use all their support and help. Heck, maybe one of them will want to join you in the process. Many times, when one person gets up the gumption to embark on a journey like this, they inspire others around them to do it, too. My husband is almost always willing to join me in a new health routine, usually a way of eating or an exercise regimen.

And finally, visualize the win. Visualization is one of the most useful techniques very successful people use to win, whether in business or athletics. Add a couple of minutes to your daily schedule to close your eyes and visualize the person you plan to become. See yourself there. See how you interact with others. See yourself standing there talking to someone. Visualize achieving your goal. Doing this daily is huge!

Commit: Write Down Your BodyWork Option

Ok! You are at the end of the BodyWork section. What have you learned? Did you change your mind as you were planning?

It's time to commit to your choice and write it down if you haven't already.

I know you are going to do well because you have gotten this far in the book. Keep your BodyWork option in the forefront of your mind as we delve into BrainWork. You're gonna love this!

PART THREE

BRAINWORK

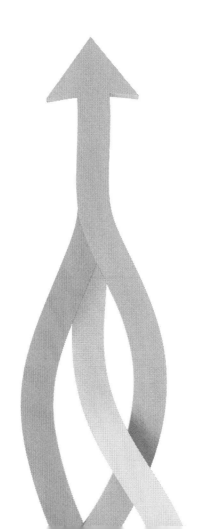

CHAPTER 7

The Brain's Role in Longevity

Your vision will become clear only when you can look into your own heart. Who looks outside, dreams; who looks inside, awakes.
— CARL JUNG

BrainWork is about the mind, the emotions, the soul, the spirit, memory, trauma, and all those complicated and unseen areas.

How does BrainWork help you live a longer, healthier life? Remember the longevity studies mentioned earlier? They talked about such things as following your intuition, releasing suppressed emotions, spirituality, and stress, all of which are related to BrainWork.

Your Mind Is a Tool

Developing your mind is critical in your pursuit of wellness and longevity. Just as our bodies speak to us through physical symptoms, our minds speak to us through thoughts, feelings, and mental symptoms. Thinking of our minds as tools can help us gain more knowledge and take more control to make better progress in all areas of our health.

You can use your mind to benefit you in so many ways. Here are some:

Interpreting your body's signals. When your body speaks, learn what it is telling you. You have to practice this like any other skill. It requires mindfulness and listening to your intuition.

Many people automatically shut off signals they don't understand. You might have to retrain yourself to stop doing that. Listen to what your body is saying. It is your inner guide. Trust it.

Processing emotions and trauma. In addition, your emotions must be processed. You probably know this by now, but it can still be difficult to do and easy to avoid. Grief, anger, resentment, trauma, fear, anxiety, etc. — we need to feel them, understand them, and then let them move through and out of our bodies.

Creating more for yourself. Your mind can create better health and more opportunities. Remember, garbage in, garbage out. If you put bad things in through your senses (eyes, ears, mouth, etc.), bad things (words, emotions, feelings, actions, poor physical and mental health) will result.

What goes into your mind affects your mental and emotional health. If your inner dialogue is negative, your mind will believe it. If you speak positively to yourself, your mind will believe that, too. Which will serve you more?

Creating a better sense of connection and purpose. Seek God in whatever way you view that. Read, listen, watch, meditate, pray. Get into nature. Go on a retreat. Go to church. Talk about it with others. This will also help you find purpose in life, deal with difficult situations, and give you hope and a more optimistic view of life. More on this when we get to WorldWork.

Releasing Deep Trauma

The unexamined life is not worth living.
— SOCRATES

Remember my friend Gail and how she was so attracted to the lavender oil that helped with her hormones? One day, she found out why — and the reason shocked her.

She was paging through a book that explained emotions, their connection to physical issues, and which essential oils help them. She learned that lavender was connected to three different emotions, one of which was abandonment.

Stunned, she had to read that section again as the pieces started falling together. She had done enough personal development and therapy over the years to know full well that abandonment was a vital issue for her. Her struggle was rooted in the horrible experience of sexual abuse she'd had as a child. In a child's mind, parents are there to keep the child safe. Unfortunately, things can happen beyond parents' control, and this was the case with Gail's situation. Still, the child in Gail, who didn't understand the complexities of the situation, felt as if she'd been abandoned, regardless of whether it was anyone's intention or fault.

During Gail's first marriage, her fear of abandonment created difficulties. "I was very co-dependent," she told me. Her husband, who had his own problems, eventually had an affair. He didn't show up to marriage counseling.

After going to counseling for a while by herself, Gail realized she had to leave the marriage and that her relationship with God was the only place she could get what she needed emotionally and spiritually. She recalls this was the worst and best day of her life — the worst because this marriage in which she had her three precious babies was over, and yet the best because she was finding God.

As she started healing, she began to take care of herself more — "loving myself more," as she puts it. Her energy levels increased, and her life started looking up.

The body part associated with abandonment is the small intestine. That is also the area around the menstrual pain Gail had at times, which the lavender helped. Gail also remembers that while growing up, she had a very sensitive digestive system — another sign of the mind/body connection.

Abandonment issues still pop up for Gail from time to time, but she knows how to handle her stress response. She may remember the affirmation associated with abandonment, "I embrace all of life's experiences," and say that to herself several times, calming herself. She may also be moved to pray. She has developed good practices that help her move through the situation calmly.

The Only Way Out Is Through

Understanding yourself, your triggers, your background, and your trauma is critical. And we all have different types and degrees of trauma.

Even something as simple as a troubling dialogue with someone can leave scars.

Understanding yourself, your triggers, your background, and your trauma is critical.

We must work through those issues to come out on the other side. You have probably heard the phrase, "The only way out is through." I know we don't want it to be true, but darn it, it is.

As for me, I experienced the trauma of rape at knifepoint by a stranger breaking into my home in the middle of the night when I lived in San Antonio, Texas. It was 1984, and I was 23 years old, living in my first apartment by myself.

At age 30, I finally went to therapy for it. Emotionally, it felt like I might die if I had to talk about it, but rationally, I knew this was ridiculous and got my courage up to do it.

A few hours of that kind of therapy moved mountains for me. I could not ignore, forget about, or go around the experience. I had to go through it, talk about every aspect — even relive it in a therapeutic setting — and then embrace it as part of who I am.

Sorting through these emotions is like peeling an onion, layer by layer. Over time, we understand more and more of who we are. Even if we've done this kind of work, it is important to continue through our lives. And we really aren't done until we die. Don't you want to feel equipped to handle this part of your life? I know I do.

Stress Takes a Toll

Nervousness and a quickening heartbeat during stressful situations are part of a physiological stress response. Two things happen: Your brain releases hormones, and your adrenal glands release cortisol. This response is good in occasional emergency situations. It is called the "fight or flight" response, and it activates to give your body the energy to save you from threats.

However, if you, like most people in our modern world, are under chronic stress every day, the resulting cascade of hormones and neurochemicals can have a profound, detrimental effect on your immune system.

This is why we must engage in stress-reducing activities like meditation, deep breathing, long baths, getting into nature, and exercise. These activities and others immediately lower our stress response.

When chronically stressed, you are more prone to viral infections, wound healing takes longer, cancer growth speeds up, and aging speeds up. Even if stress is not necessarily causing these (they can be caused by other factors), stress definitely speeds up all of the effects.

Our Thoughts and Words Can Create Our Situation

Here's a great example of how mindset affects health.

In 1981, Dodie Osteen, the mother of Joel Osteen, pastor of Lakewood Church in Houston, Texas, was informed by her doctor that she had metastatic cancer of the liver and had weeks to live.

All her life, she had been the picture of health. In fact, she recounts saying often, "I am disgustingly healthy." She does not say that anymore. Not because she is not healthy but because she knows the power of our words and will never take her health for granted again.

With no hope from the medical community, her husband told the doctor that they believed in miracles and in the miracle worker (that would be Jesus), and they were going home to pray and seek God for what to do.

She is the first to say, "Do not necessarily do what I did." Seek God, and do what brings peace to you. Peace is the barometer for what you need to do in any situation.

After she went home, she had many people pray for her, but one night, she felt she heard God speak to her heart, "Dodie, others' faith will not heal you. It is YOUR faith that you must go on now." She knew at that point that it was between her and Jesus.

Therefore, she began to live as if she were not sick. She felt awful but knew it would only get worse if she stayed in bed. She forced herself to continue to operate as best she could — taking no naps, sleeping the normal number of hours at night, and praying fervently. She prayed daily, in first person, forty specific Bible verses relating to her health.

To make a long story short — she didn't die. In fact, she got healthier. Did she go back for tests to confirm her health? No. She knew she was healthy. She didn't want hospital tests messing with her faith.

A few years later, she saw a doctor about another issue, and they reported that she was as healthy as a young woman. Her doctors, well-known in medicine, say the only explanation is that she had healed supernaturally. Her story is in her book called *Healed of Cancer.*[59]

How is your mindset? What words do you hear yourself speaking in your mind to yourself? Are you kind to yourself? Do you choose words of life? Words that are positive and uplifting?

Sometimes, we must make ourselves speak a certain way to get it to anchor into our brains. There is a saying that some love and others do not. "Fake it till you make it." I think this is a good saying. Sometimes, we need to speak things that we may not actually believe yet, even though we want to, but as time goes on, and the more we say it, we do start to believe it.

It really requires awareness to notice how you speak in the quietness of your mind. These words will typically come out of your mouth too. This includes good things or bad.

> *It really requires awareness to notice how you speak in the quietness of your mind. These words will typically come out of your mouth too.*

Science Shows Us the Effects of Our Words

In his book *Messages in Water,* Dr. Masuru Emoto from Japan demonstrates the importance of the words we speak.

He studied the effects on water of exposing it to certain words and then freezing it.

The water that was exposed to loving, beautiful words formed into perfect crystal structures. The water exposed to hateful, unkind words formed into nonsymmetrical, distorted, and ugly structures.[60]

This is a fascinating study and will give you a good visual (a quick online search will show you the pictures) when you think about your words and thoughts and the effect they have on your body or on other people. (Remember, the body is mostly made up of water.)

Choose your words wisely.

In the biblical book of wisdom, Proverbs 18:21 (NKJV) says, "Death and life is in the power of the tongue and those who love it will eat its fruit." Or, in another version (MSG), "Words kill, words give life. They're either poison or fruit — you choose."

Healing through Spirituality

This is a tricky topic because there are so many different religious and spiritual beliefs. I would ask you to remain open-minded and try not to let certain words trigger you.

A spiritual connection, community, or practice is listed in the longevity studies, but what does that mean?

One concept I have heard and believed for quite a while is this: We are a spirit, we have a soul (mind, will, and emotions), and we live in a body.

We are a spirit, we have a soul (mind, will, and emotions), and we live in a body.

Someone who believes we are simply a physical body without the other parts will probably just search for physical solutions to illness or longevity in general without pursuing the other avenues of mind and spirit.

According to Dr. Turner, author of *Radical Remission*:

> *A spiritual practice is one that encourages you to feel — in your body and your emotions — a deep sensation of calm and peace. In order to feel this, you first have to find a way to shut off your thinking mind.*
>
> *Many people feel spiritual energy very subtly at first, like a gentle wave of calmness — the way you might feel after watching a sunset. If you want to intensify that post-sunset feeling, you will likely have to commit to doing your spiritual practice daily so the feeling can build up over time. ...*
>
> *When the thinking mind stops, and spiritual energy begins to flow through you, a whole host of healthy changes occur in your physical body, including a rush of healthy hormones streaming from your pineal and pituitary glands into your bloodstream, increased oxygenation of the body, improved blood circulation, decreased blood pressure, improved digestion and detoxification, a stronger immune system, and the ability to turn off unhealthy genes.* [61]

More good motivation!

People find their method of spiritual connection in different ways. The important thing is to find what works for you and do it daily. For those who practice daily for a short period, that spiritual connection can last all day. If the practice is sporadic because we are too busy, that connection can be weak and difficult to maintain, leading to a general lack of peace in life and possibly even disease.

A study documented in Science Direct found that practicing meditation produces high levels of melatonin in the body.[62] I love that! We should definitely meditate before going to bed if we have issues in that department.

Turner also states that, according to another Pub Med study, "meditating for thirty minutes a day for eight weeks decreases the density of your brain areas associated with anxiety and stress and increases your brain matter density in the areas associated with empathy and memory."[63]

Pitfalls to Avoid

Don't Own a Diagnosis

Make sure you don't verbally own or identify yourself with any particular diagnosis. Once again, your words are crucial to your body's healing. What you think comes out of your mouth. You have thoughts, and then words are created. Changing your thoughts is key and very possible. This is what we were doing earlier with the affirmations.

If you say things like "my cancer," "my cold," "my diabetes," or anything else like that, we know the thoughts inside your head believe that malady **belongs** to you. It's no longer JUST a diagnosis someone else gave you — someone who doesn't know the relationship between you and your creator.

So, give that person who gave you a diagnosis, or the words that person spoke, or the words in the report no power over you. Instead, regardless of what the report says, you can say something like, "The report said diabetes. My body is healing wonderfully every day." Or even better, you could choose not to say the diagnosis word at all. I have an acquaintance who has successfully fought cancer using a few modern and many natural processes. Instead of calling it cancer, she calls it "sushi." I love that.

Don't own the disease. You're not lying. You're choosing to speak words of life. If the people around you think that's weird, then don't talk about it with them. Make sense?

To drill this in even more, don't call it "my" unless you love having it. It is way too much for your brain to have to overcome.

> *Don't own the disease. You're not lying. You're choosing to speak words of life. If the people around you think that's weird, then don't talk about it with them.*

You may not believe these words you speak right now, but over time, when you speak the correct words, you will. And when you do, I believe your body and your brain will work better together in your healing process.

Negativity Creates Stagnation

Some people don't try to figure out their lives — who they are, where they came from, why they do the things they do. Years of negative programming have likely created this.

Does this sound like you? If so, you may need to purposely pursue self-understanding, even though you don't naturally want to.

If low self-esteem is involved, make sure you are in some kind of counseling and surround yourself with uplifting people. You will need to work at believing in yourself. You can absolutely do this. It just may take some time and consistency.

Maybe you have pursued personal development before, but it just didn't work out for some reason. Hey, try again! It can take a while to find your path in this area.

Remember — take baby steps. You may not know where you are headed, and that may create some negativity, but one step will lead to another, even if you don't know what that next step is. I got into that calendar, which led me to 75 Hard, which led me to a women's mastermind, which led me to the idea of writing a book. All those steps were unknowns. I just kept plugging along, sensing inside that it was heading somewhere important.

As you get into the next section of this book, you will be reconnecting with your special gifts, skills, and talents. Sometimes, we disconnect with them because we have spent so many years focused on taking care of others, whether our children and family or our jobs. Getting back to the special way we were created can give us an injection of energy and excitement for our future.

We all have a story, we all have dysfunction in our families, we all have areas that we think are broken or just don't work. We are human, imperfect, and messy. It's all good, my friend. This is the beauty of life. Hang in there!

Is Time Moving Too Fast?

Claudia Hammond, a psychologist and BBC columnist, tells about this concept in *Scientific American*.[64] Our brain puts many similar moments of our life together as if it's one memory. These are the things we do the same day after day. That is why it's easy to wonder, "Where did this year go?"

Meanwhile, when we do new and different things (i.e., get out of our comfort zone), our brain stores those as separate memories, which in turn makes time feel longer. This is why when we were children and experiencing new things all the time, time felt longer. The same occurs when we travel and have new experiences.

It's our choice as to whether our life feels long or if it feels like it speeds by in the blink of an eye. The more we are on autopilot, the faster time seems to go. So, let's get out of that comfort zone, whether in our minds or in our physical activities and strive for longevity — whether in actual years or in the feeling of time going by in our minds.

Self-Reflection: Where Are You with BrainWork?

Do you ever sit quietly with a pen and paper and just randomly start writing your thoughts, allowing your pen to go where it wants without any kind of censor in your brain telling you what not to write?

Have you ever written out the story of any trauma you have experienced?

Have you added the idea of a brain download to your routine? Do you start your day by writing out everything on your mind?

Have you taken any personality tests over the years? Which ones? Do you think it might be beneficial to take some?

Have you ever read any personal development books? Which subjects would you like to explore more?

If you have a business, are there personal development books you want to read about how you can be a better leader?

Do you prefer to listen to audiobooks or podcasts? They exist on every subject you can think of. What subject would you like to explore in this way?

Whether you are a Christian or not, have you read the Bible? The whole thing? Is that something you would like to do?

Are there any other spiritually oriented books you would like to read or that you think would benefit your mindset and spiritual connection?

How do you feel about the environments you spend the most time in? For most people, these are probably the bedroom, bathroom, kitchen, living room, office, and car. How would you rate your satisfaction with these environments? Are they cluttered or streamlined? Do you think working on these areas would help your mindset?

Do you ever spend time in meditation or prayer? Do you think this would be beneficial to your life? Do you know how to do these?

How is your stress level? How do you de-stress? Do you want to find more ways to lower your stress level?

Do you think including any of these in your Sixty-Day Dare would be beneficial?

Which ones and why?

Now that you're thinking about these things let's explore the BrainWork Big Five.

CHAPTER 8

The BrainWork Big Five

Talk to yourself like you would to someone you love.
— BRENÉ BROWN

Like the BodyWork Big Five, the BrainWork Big Five were created with the most important findings from the research we've already looked at. These BrainWork Big Five options are:

- **WRITE** – Write at least 10 minutes a day. Journal, brain download, etc.
- **READ** – Read at least 10 pages a day in your non-fiction book, or spend an equivalent length of time with an uplifting audiobook or podcast.

- **CLEAR** – Do at least 15 minutes a day of decluttering or detoxing your home to declutter and clear your mind and to create a home without toxic chemicals.
- **MEDITATE** – Pray, meditate, or do affirmations for at least 10 minutes a day.
- **CREATE** – Devote at least 30 minutes a day to your creative endeavor.

Why These Five?

Anyone who has done research into how we help ourselves in areas such as releasing suppressed emotions, uplifting ourselves, lowering our stress level, or learning new things knows that these areas are the top activities to engage in. They are often recommended by therapists, and if you search online, these will come up over and over.

Plus, I know from personal experience that they work. I have been practicing these off and on for decades. They have helped me tremendously, and I know they will help you too.

Let's explore them in more detail to help you pick the best option.

#1: WRITE – Guidelines and Ideas

Writing can be very therapeutic, and you can use it in several ways. Here are some ways to do the Write option:

Daily Journaling. Simply journal daily about your life, desires, prayers, and concerns. You can also journal to help release any trauma story you have in your past. Are there traumatic experiences in your life that you've kept to yourself for years, even decades? We all have them. Start writing them out. That process will start the healing. And remember, your journal is for no one else to read. This type of journaling might be something you choose to keep or not. You decide.

Morning Pages. I learned about these in the 90s from Julia Cameron in her book *The Artist's Way.*[65] It consists of producing three pages of writing, pen and paper, stream of consciousness, every morning, ideally close to the time you wake up. As you write, allow anything to come out. Sometimes, past issues come up, and other times, you are just focused on how you feel right then about what happened yesterday. If you're doing this option, you can use the three-pages measurement rather than the 10 minutes.

Stream-of-consciousness writing can give you access to your subconscious and can lead to increased creativity, insight, and more understanding of who you are.

These Morning Pages can be thrown away if you like. Sometimes, they are even nonsensical, just to keep the pen moving. Once you get things out, you will start leaving space for the future, ideas, plans, dreams, and lovely things.

Dream Diary. *Similarly, if you tend to remember your dreams, you could keep a dream diary and write about them upon waking each morning. This can be another path to knowing yourself better. Research ways to do this. This could be combined with your daily journaling or your morning pages.*

Remember, all of these are best done with pen and paper. Writing with your hand has brain benefits. (Another fun topic to research!)

#2: READ – Guidelines and Ideas

The reading I'm talking about here is non-fiction for self-knowledge and building skills.

For me, it is easy to peruse a book, skip around, and just read what immediately grabs me, but one of the best things I did in 75 Hard was pick a good book, make myself sit down every day, and read the next ten pages, ultimately finishing the book. It is a fantastic practice, and it really doesn't take long. Ten pages a day is a good amount — and make sure your next book is waiting in the wings for when you finish the first.

You can also listen to an audiobook, podcast, or digital course. The goal is to consume content that will uplift or improve you in some way. If you are already a big audiobook or podcast listener, I'd recommend reading a book. Following are some ideas for subjects, but you can pick something else as long as it meets the requirements.

Know Yourself. One excellent start to gain that deep self-understanding is to do a good personality test. These can help you understand why you do what you do, why other people in your life do what they do, and how you can interact with others in a healthier way.

It can not only enhance your understanding of yourself and maybe even your purpose on earth but can transform your marriage or a relationship with your child, a sibling, or anyone close to you. It can also improve your work life.

One of the best tests I've ever done, and I've done a lot, is the Enneagram. It categorizes people into nine types based on childhood wounds. This system definitely goes deep. It looks at the inner motivation that leads to your behaviors and then provides a path to healing. Multiple authors have written about it. My favorite is Ian Morgan Cron and his book *The Road Back to You.*[66] He also has a podcast called *Typology.*[67]

Reading about the Enneagram has probably helped my marriage more than anything. Understanding how The Individualist (me) and The Helper (my husband) can get along better has been incredibly helpful over the years.

If you choose this option, first do the test and then find the materials to read about your type. With some tests, you can also go online to find forums and interact with others of your particular type to learn how they deal with things you might be facing too.

Uplift. This is another option for reading or listening to material, but it is focused on increasing positive emotions or spiritual connection. It might be a podcast on some aspect of natural health or maybe a sermon or an interview on a spiritual subject. It might be an audiobook. It might also be an autobiography about someone you admire.

You can listen while you're doing so many other things. I listen while I walk, putter around the house, prep my Airbnb for the next guest, put makeup on, garden, or get into bed at night.

Learn or Build Skills. Building skills stimulates your brain, creating more neural pathways and neuroplasticity.

All things that lead to longevity. Again, the idea here is to better yourself.

If you are an entrepreneur or you are working on your purpose or mission, this can include books or podcasts on how to be a better leader or how to do anything that improves key areas.

You might want to read or listen to the subjects of marketing your ideas or your product and how to do that better. Maybe you are trying to hire key people and need to up your skills in the recruiting and hiring department. What are the key questions to ask someone? How could you conduct a better interview? Maybe you need to learn how to speak in front of an audience.

Or maybe you want to develop new creative skills, so you need to read about how to knit a sweater, how to design a garden, or which plants work well with others in zone 7.

The sky is the limit on building skills, and searching for books that appeal to you is such a fun endeavor.

#3: CLEAR – Guidelines and Ideas

In this section, you can choose to declutter your home or clear it of toxic products in favor of natural, chemical-free choices.

Declutter. Disorganized spaces can trigger stress and anxiety. Decluttering and organizing your environment can bring you peace of mind and clarity. It can improve your sleep, help with focus and concentration, assist with better eating habits, and simplify taking care of your home. Essentially, it helps your overall mental and physical health.

Yes, we are back to "environment triggers behavior." We want our environment to trigger good things in our brain, which trigger good things in our behavior.

If you choose to declutter your house or even a single room, it can feel overwhelming. Instead, why not try a different approach? One of my favorite books on decluttering is Marie Kondo's *The Life-Changing Magic of Tidying Up*.[68] In it, she uses the technique of decluttering by item type. For instance, decluttering your short-sleeved shirts. First, you get every short-sleeved shirt you own and lay it on your bed. The ones in your closet, the ones in your drawers, the ones in that other closet... get them all out. You need to see them all at once.

Then, start sorting. You can probably do a first run-through and pull out several to throw in the donation pile or trash. Have a box for each category nearby. On your next go-around, you may need to get more specific — split them into sections of dressy tops, T-shirts, business tops, etc., and then assess each group to see what to keep or get rid of.

Only keep what brings you joy and/or what is truly functional. It's hard to get rid of things you've spent good money on, but sending that article of clothing out to someone else who WILL love it will bring you good spiritual energy, and it will also help eliminate those bad feelings you have for not ever wearing it. (I'm talking to myself here too.)

One time, I got ruthless with my closet and kept only eight outfits. I was at the height of mothering and schooling all five children at home, and I needed my life super-simplified. I'll never forget how incredible it felt to have only those eight outfits — enough for one each day, plus one extra. My closet was so clean and streamlined. You don't have to go to those lengths, but I promise you will feel so much better once you tackle this.

Another way to focus is in small sections. For instance, you could do one kitchen drawer per session or a different area of your living room each session. You can even just time yourself in an area — for instance, set a timer and devote 30 minutes a day to decluttering that location.

If you really want to feel motivated and make huge progress in decluttering, do what I do and play Kondo's audiobook while you are going through the process. Something about her voice helps get me through it and motivates me.

Another tool I love is the Netflix series called Home Edit.[69] Two ladies go into houses and completely organize a room. It will inspire you and teach you what tools will help you do the same. They have books with the same name.[70]

Detoxify. On the subject of detoxing your home, think back to Gail and how all of those products full of chemicals (many of which are banned in Europe) were disrupting her endocrine system. Switching these (cleaners, shampoos, skincare products, soaps, makeup, etc.) with non-toxic ones can make a huge difference in your health, and it's so easy to do.

Most of this work will happen in your bathrooms, kitchen, and laundry room, and wherever else you have your cosmetics/personal-care items (car or purse, workplace desk, etc.). This is a process. Just take it room by room (or area by area).

The big thing to remember is that in the U.S., there are trade secrets, and companies do not have to tell us the ingredients in their products. So, if you cannot see what the ingredients are, that is a good sign that they are not good, and you should steer away from them. Companies that use healthy ingredients will promote that fact. Here is a good start on which items you should be making sure are toxin- and chemical-free.

Bathroom – Toothpaste, mouthwash, floss, shampoo, conditioner, soap, lotion, skin care products, deodorant, lip balm, makeup, perfume (use high-grade essential oils instead).

Bedroom – Get rid of candles. Use essential oil diffusers instead. Bedding and mattresses. Use natural, 100-percent cotton or linen sheets.

Laundry Room – Laundry soap (Note: add baking soda and vinegar to your healthy laundry soap for heavy-duty jobs). Get rid of dryer sheets. Use wool balls with drops of essential oils on them instead.

Kitchen – Dish soap, hand soap, pot scrub, dishwasher detergent, rinse aid (use citric acid instead).

Lifestyle – Sunscreen, after-sun skin care, insect repellent, cough drops, energy drinks, energy shots, pain cream, sports gel, protein powder, vitamins and supplements.

Devote a certain amount of time each day to researching, purchasing, making "homemade," and setting up your home with natural products. Beware of greenwashing. Some companies make dubious or false claims about their product's environmental impact to mislead consumers. Read labels. Know what is in your products, or find people you trust who do.

> *Beware of greenwashing. Some companies make dubious or false claims about their product's environmental impact to mislead consumers. Read labels.*

#4: MEDITATE – Guidelines and Ideas

This section includes meditation, prayer, and affirmations. If you feel you have a high degree of stress in your life, or if you have been wanting to do this but haven't set aside the time, this may be the one for you. Devoting ten or twenty minutes a day to meditation, prayer, or affirmations for sixty days could dramatically change your life.

Meditation. The word meditation has caused confusion among Christians over the years. Don't let semantics take you off course — you can meditate and still follow scripture. The Bible tells us to meditate or contemplate on scriptures or God's attributes. The word "meditate" just means "focus on."

By closing your eyes, you can focus on your breathing as you inhale and exhale. You can focus on counting. You can focus on certain scriptures or certain affirmations that speak to you. Even scripture in the form of affirmations can be wonderful.

You can listen to guided meditations that uphold your beliefs. There are many available. The point is to learn to focus and quiet the mind. To reduce stress, anxiety, and depression. To gain deeper insights. To anchor us in love. Meditating allows us to shift out of fight or flight and get back in control.

Prayer. Talk to God in whatever way works for you. If you are not used to doing that, it can feel weird and awkward, but that's okay; just do it weirdly and awkwardly. He is totally fine with that. Talk to Him like a best friend. If you're angry, tell Him why. He doesn't get offended.

Instead of phrasing it as a future-oriented request, I really like praying by starting with "Thank you" as if the thing I hope for has already happened. I like to believe that on the spiritual plane, there really is no such thing as time. This actually combines prayer and affirmations.

For example, I would say, "Thank you, God, that my children seek You and find You," versus praying, "God, I pray my children will seek and find You." See the difference? That word "will" puts things off into the future. I want this now, and I know my words manifest into things. Thoughts turn into words. Words manifest into the physical world. So, I want to speak as if the thing is done.

I'm thanking Him that it is already done and believe that it is, in fact, done on the spiritual plane and just needs to manifest on earth now. It makes me think of the verse, "On earth, as it is in heaven." This may sound woo-woo, but it is how my brain works best. And, always, of course, "His will be done."

Affirmations. Affirmations are positive, "I am" or "I do" statements used to combat negative thinking. Pub Med research from the University of Wisconsin showed that MRI evidence suggests that some neural pathways are increased by self-affirmation.[71]

Affirmations, like everything else in this chapter, require continuous use to make a difference. Come up with some key affirmations that apply to your life, set aside time to focus on them, and repeat them to yourself several times. One idea would be to read your affirmations once in the morning and once at night, totaling the amount of time needed for the 10-minute goal. You can divide the time with a longer session in the morning and shorter at night, depending on your needs.

Here are a few examples I like from mindset coach Dena Patton:

- "I own my authenticity, my goals, my faith, and my gifts without apology."
- "I am comfortable with upholding my boundaries and saying no."
- "I create and maintain powerful daily systems, boundaries, and structures to achieve my goals."

Try saying them aloud. Doesn't it make you feel good?

You can create or find affirmations for many things, such as abundance, healing, protection, self-love, success, gratitude, creativity, clarity, spirituality, and more. Write out the ones that really speak to you and dedicate time each day to reading them. Eventually, you will probably have them memorized.

#5: CREATE – Guidelines and Ideas

Are you having enough fun in your life? Do you have hobbies you love that you regularly engage in that are also creative pursuits? I believe everyone is creative, and you just have to find something that interests you.

Why is this important? At the top of the list is that a creative outlet can reduce stress. It can also enhance cognitive function. Hidden talents can emerge if given the chance. It can connect us with a new passion. It can help us think outside the box and solve problems in a new way. It can increase happiness and contentment, as well as a sense of purpose and fulfillment. That's a lot of good stuff!

It's probably no surprise to learn from a study of thirty-nine adults cited in the *Journal of the American Art Therapy Association* that just forty-five minutes of artmaking can significantly lower cortisol levels.[72] We want those levels lowered and used only for their right purposes in our bodies. Chronically high cortisol is not good for us.

This artmaking can be what we call "getting into that flow state," a beautiful thing. We women are often so busy raising babies for so many years or locked into a power career that we never really develop a good creative hobby to escape to for an hour here or there — or maybe, oh my, even a whole day!

I've already mentioned my own favorite hobby, which I discovered kind of by accident about three years ago. My mother-in-law was a master needlepointer, and she made my children and me gorgeous Christmas stockings over the years. By the time child number five came along, she could no longer do it. I thought, "Oh my goodness, I'm going to have to make this child a needlepoint stocking that can measure up to these other works of art because they will be side by side forever!"

I had done very small needlepoint projects a few times over the years, but I was not that into it. I searched and finally found a gorgeous canvas stocking for her and proceeded to work on it a little each year for about eight years. Good grief. Eventually, I thought, I MUST get this finished before she gets any older, so that year, I worked on it constantly. And guess what happened?

I got addicted to it. It became a total stress reducer for me. I love going to the shops now, watching people talk about it online, searching for beautiful canvases, feeling the silk and wool threads in my fingers, and creating something beautiful that will become an heirloom for my children. I can do larger pieces at home, and I can travel with smaller ones.

As I mentioned, it is my reward for a good, productive day of work, and I look soooooo forward to it. Currently, after I spend about two to six hours daily focused on writing this book, plus all the other random tasks of the day, my reward is to retreat to my chair and needlepoint while listening to something uplifting or watching my latest binge TV series. Yes, the TV is my guilty pleasure! My rationalization is that I used to work in TV, and I love the art of filmmaking. Also, I'm good at rationalizing things!

I WILL say that it required me to engage in needlepoint as often as I could for it to become a desirable habit. I was determined to get that thing done. So, if you are looking to develop a new creative outlet or habit, give yourself grace as you pursue it for your sixty days and become more proficient.

One more point: Do not confuse this activity for your Sixty-Day Dare with the WorldWork mission/ purpose or calling. Yes, it may very well be that your work is a creative art you love where you get into that flow state, and it is a stress reducer. However, if it is also your mission in life and you have goals to achieve with it, that may put a different spin on it. The production, marketing, and selling of it may change the nature of it simply being a stress reducer. We'll get more into that in the next section.

Commit: Write Down Your BrainWork Choice

It's time to decide where you want to start. Get out your notebook, planner, or app, and write down your choice. If you haven't decided yet, just take some notes on which of these areas you would like to pursue and why. As you start planning in the next chapter, you will begin to nail it down. Do not fear. It is going to be awesome!

CHAPTER 9

Planning Your BrainWork

Change is inevitable. Growth is optional.
— JOHN C. MAXWELL

I hope you've written down your option for your BrainWork Big Five or have at least narrowed down your thoughts some. In this chapter, our job is to integrate your choices from BodyWork with your choices in BrainWork and make sure you are set up for success.

Before we go a second further, one critical subject we women must discuss is boundaries. This affects all three areas of BodyWork, BrainWork, and WorldWork, but it is located here in the BrainWork section because boundaries require our minds to create them and make them stick. If we don't do this, we will most likely not be successful in following through with our Sixty-Day Dare.

Set Your Own Boundaries

Being a woman, not to mention a mother, is hard work. Because of our nature, we tend to put others first, mostly our children. While admirable, taken too far, this quality becomes detrimental. It is unhealthy for both you and the focus of your time and energy, which could be anything from a loved one to a job or an organization.

How are you at setting boundaries with others and keeping them? In other words, how are you at teaching people how to treat you?

Yes, it's true: We teach people how to treat us. This is the difference between having a victim mindset versus an accountability mindset. Whether you're defining physical or emotional boundaries, the definition begins with your mental focus.

We teach people how to treat us.

Being a Victim Versus Being Accountable

Accountability does not imply situations like crimes or abuse are the victim's fault. I'm not trying to shame victims — they are not responsible for someone else's actions. What I want you to know about is a small mindset shift that can help *prevent* you from living with a victim mindset.

It's about how you look at your life. While you can't control others' actions, you are the only one who can create the life you desire. No one else will do it for you. This can be a rude awakening.

Thankfully, I learned this lesson while I was in my twenties, less than a year after the assault in my apartment. I had agreed to attend a weekend personal development seminar that a friend recommended. During one exercise, the program leaders asked the seventy participants to remember a time we felt we were victims.

Oh, my. I couldn't think of anything other than the assault. Tears started streaming down my face.

They asked us to take off those victim-viewing glasses we were looking at that situation through and change them to a different pair of glasses — an accountability-viewing pair. How did we possibly contribute to that situation, and how could we be responsible for it?

What the hell? I *was* a victim. How could I be accountable? Ugh.

I decided to come up with some answers and play the game, even though I didn't believe I would learn anything I didn't already know.

My answers surprised me.

For instance, I had haphazardly left the curtains on my sliding glass door barely parted, allowing anyone to see in. I hadn't made sure the door was locked that evening. Even my choice of apartment was an issue. I had accepted an apartment at the back of the complex near an alley, where random construction workers were working daily.

Though I was a victim of a crime that night, that exercise made me realize that I hadn't done enough to protect myself in the first place. And, of course, I started to think about how I could prevent something like that in the future.

The ability to consider all aspects of a circumstance, even though I might not have been at fault, stayed with me over the next four decades and solidified my desire to not ever consider myself a victim regardless of the situation. I certainly wouldn't wish that horrible experience on anyone, but always looking at the world through a lens of accountability has been one of the best skills I could have asked for. It *is* a skill, and anyone can develop it.

That was an extreme example, but here is a seemingly minor example that is oh, so common. I would love it if you got rid of the statement "I don't have time" and instead started saying, "It's not a priority right now." That is being accountable versus being a victim of time. It is also the truth. We all have the same amount of time. We prioritize what is most important. Decide what you will prioritize and then speak accordingly.

You Can Say No

Let me preface this by saying, obviously, I'm not talking about extreme situations where you literally have no choice. What I mean is that if someone is treating you badly, they are responsible for their own actions, but you may have also allowed it in some way. It really is that simple.

That may be tough to hear, but it's true. It all goes back to boundaries. What are you willing to tolerate? What are you not willing to tolerate? What kind of protection are you willing to give yourself? How can you be vigilant about meeting your own needs?

If your boundaries are blurry, I recommend therapy or some co-dependent group sessions to understand better. The book *Boundaries* by Henry Cloud[73] is a good one to read.

It is never too late to set boundaries. We grow, we change, and it's perfectly fine to say to someone, "Hey, you know, I've just realized that this thing is really important in my life, and I have to make some changes. So, I won't be able to do that thing anymore. Thanks so much for understanding." You'll know that person really cares if they can hear your heart and be okay with it.

The bottom line is you must carve out time and set boundaries with others to get healthy, stay healthy, and pursue your dreams. Sometimes, it is just all about saying no. I know many of us find it very hard to say no — but you must.

Your Purpose Is on The Line

When you say yes to what someone else wants, you are saying no to something else — something that may be vitally important to you, your health, your dreams, or your purpose. The reason God sent you here. Maybe you don't even know what it is, but you need time and room to explore it.

One of my favorite sayings lately is, "Leave room for the magic." If we are so busy helping everyone else, we have left no room for ourselves to figure things out.

> *Leave room for the magic.*

You also need to set this example for your children, whether they are grown or not. They need to see their parents pursuing their dreams so they will do the same thing. The world needs everyone's gifts.

Get over That Mom-Guilt! (And Yes, I Know It's Hard)

One of my most significant boundary-setting moments was about eight years ago. I was 55 and had hit one of those thresholds. I'd been homeschooling our children for 17 years at that point. I loved the responsibility of their education. Still, it was heavy, and feeling young and invincible, I put my own health on the back burner.

After reading a book on exercising in one's later years, I vividly remember saying to myself, "I am going to start exercising consistently no matter what. No matter if my children never get educated. No matter if they are wearing crappy clothes or eating cereal for dinner. I am going to keep my health because if I'm dead, ain't no one here to be the mother." It's like the flight emergency instructions: Put your own oxygen mask on first and then help the others.

Sometimes, I have to take it that far in my mind in order to commit to it. And commit I did. I began to arrange my entire life around those workouts. Though I only did a couple a week at the beginning. I didn't budge on the commitment. These children would be fine. And they were.

If someone — even my husband — wants me to do something when my workout is scheduled, the answer is no. That's because there is always a reason to skip that workout or do something different.

You need to draw these lines in the sand, too. Just say no. If you don't, you will end up physically and/or mentally sick, exhausted, anxiety-ridden, and full of regret at the end of your life.

Find a way. Because, again — the world needs you.

Now, let's think about the Four Cs to help you integrate your choices for BrainWork and BodyWork.

Be Curious: Let Your Brain Take the Lead

BrainWork is the perfect place to focus on your curiosity — after all, curiosity starts in your mind! So, it's time to think. Are there things you've been wanting to explore? Topics or activities that sound interesting? This is your time to go for that.

Are you curious about who you are and why you do what you do? Now is your time to figure this out.

If you aren't sure what you need, tell your brain to get curious about that! Take a spiritual approach: Ask God, your higher power of choice, or even your intuition to help you choose what you most need right now.

What you learn might surprise you. Here's a great example of that.

The "Why" Technique

At one point, I felt I needed more peace, and I thought my solution was to sit and meditate and journal to de-stress. However, I got curious and asked myself why I was stressed. What came up was, "Because this wall in my office stresses me out." My wall-to-wall, floor-to-ceiling bookcase was a disordered, cluttered mess of books and junk that I hated to look at.

So, instead of meditating, I went into declutter mode and tackled that bookshelf. I reordered all the books by color — blue, red, white, black, yellow — all lined up. Then, I added several shelves of white-backed magazine-type holders for all my health-related documents. Every time I look at that bookshelf now, I feel at peace. I love that I took the time to declutter it. What a difference asking "why" made! If I hadn't done that, I'd probably be meditating and still stressed, wondering why meditating wasn't helping.

This is a perfect example of how the "Why" technique can help you get to the root causes of an issue and help you decide the best way to pursue your BrainWork (or any of the categories). Continue to ask yourself "why" until you find it. Let's look at another example:

I have a lot of stress, and maybe I should start journaling about it every day.

Why?

I seem to be irritated often and overreact negatively to family members.

Why?

I don't have enough time in my day to do some things that I really want to do and I'm mad about it.

Why?

I really want to work on my poetry writing because it makes me feel so good and like I'm really accomplishing something wonderful.

Well! Now, we have arrived at the real answer. Instead of "write," as journaling, this person should probably pick "create" and focus on her poetry. I bet her family will be happy about how happy she is!

Be Creative: Make It Fun/Efficient

Let's talk about how to make each of the BrainWork Big Five more fun and more doable. I always say, if it isn't fun, then why are we doing it? Of course, there are things we must do that are not fun, but still. It's a line that makes me happy!

If it isn't fun, then why are we doing it?

Combine Self-Enhancing BodyWork and BrainWork Activities

I love "killing two birds with one stone." I think it was raising and homeschooling five children that made me really good at it. I find it almost impossible to just sit and listen to or watch a podcast or program without doing something else at the same time.

If you're like me, you're probably already thinking about that with your Sixty-Day Dare. Here are some ideas.

Let's say your BodyWork choice is to walk every day, and your BrainWork choice is to read or listen to uplifting or educational material. Those are easy to do at the same time.

You could also listen to material from podcasts or audiobooks while cooking your healthy dinners.

Suppose you decide to get a certain number of steps in per day for BodyWork. You could certainly combine that with clearing clutter in your home for BrainWork. I know when I'm in declutter mode, I can get a lot of steps in moving things all around the house.

Habit-Stacking

Habit-stacking is a technique where you attach a new habit to a habit you already have. Let's say you are pretty good at remembering to do your journaling in the morning, but you're not good at remembering to drink your water. You could focus on drinking the whole bottle of water during your journaling session. At the end, if you have any left, you have to finish it and go get another.

Plan and Prepare

If you will be focusing on reading, I would love for you to actually read books made of paper rather than an e-book. There is something about the wonderful tactile experience of a paper book that, in our modern world, we see less and less of. I love opening an old book and seeing what I underlined or jotted in the margins. (It's a shame that many schools don't have books anymore — just laptop computers.)

Start deciding on topics you want to read about and purchase them, or get them at the library so you are ready to go.

Will your focus be creating or clearing? What supplies or tools will you need to accomplish your goal? Make a list. Purchase anything you will need.

Find The Perfect Environment

Here we go again: Environment triggers behavior.

With almost any choice in BrainWork, you will want to choose a wonderful spot and maybe a time of day as well, so you develop that habit. Remember the Pavlov's dog experiment? [74]The Russian scientist Ivan Pavlov showed how, over time, with a repeated neutral stimulus like ringing a bell whenever food was presented, the dogs began to associate the bell with the arrival of food. Over time, you will begin to associate that spot with reading your book, writing, praying, or creating. After sixty days, you will just automatically get into the right mode when you're there.

Set up that environment. This is key to success. Find the perfect chair or area of your home. Maybe you need to rearrange some furniture. Get a good light. Put your books or writing materials nearby in a nicely arranged way. Maybe you will find an old pretty plate or tray to use. Make it inviting, so you want to go there.

Remember, changing your habits takes grit and determination, perseverance, belief in yourself, and trust in the process.

Remember, changing your habits takes grit and determination, perseverance, belief in yourself, and trust in the process.

It is not easy to take your vitamins when you hide them in the pantry cabinet. It isn't easy to go to the gym when the clothes and shoes you need to put on are stuffed in a drawer or in the back of the closet. It isn't easy to start work on an important project if your desk is strewn with papers, bills, and old coffee cups. Do the prep. Set up your environments for success.

Have Good Tools

If you decide to focus on writing, then it is really nice to have something you think is beautiful to write in. Find a pretty journal and your favorite pen. Set these in the special location where you will write each day.

Another fun thing to do is to buy a set of colored pens. Remember the old days when we bought all of our school supplies? How thrilling was that? Recall those feelings as you prepare for new and exciting experiences with your beautiful brain.

If you are looking for prayers, one of my favorite books, *Prayers That Avail Much* by Germaine Copeland[75], contains a prayer for almost every situation. Get the 25th Anniversary edition that contains all three of the original books. Many other books offer similar compilations.

You may also want to use the book *Releasing Emotional Patterns with Essential Oils.*[76] This is full of affirmations related to specific emotions and to areas of the body too. This would be a great way to work daily on shifting a pattern of thinking that is not serving you well. You will also want to get a few high-quality essential oils to inhale while doing the affirmations. This can be a wonderful, fulfilling, life-changing option.

You can also search online for affirmations having to do with a certain subject matter. Print those off and keep them in your special spot.

Get Enthusiastic About Decluttering Your World

Let's talk about *clearing* for a moment.

Just making the decision to declutter my environment gets me excited. If you choose this for your sixty days, start by making a list of areas or a type of item (clothes, for instance) you want to declutter. Also, decide on the time of day you will do it.

The Home Edit gals use this process: Edit, Contain, Maintain. [77]

Edit – Pull everything out and get rid of what you don't love or isn't functional.

Contain – Find a spot for everything. If your budget allows, you may want to purchase some containers. The Container Store is crazy fun but also a bit pricey. Amazon and those types of places, garage sales, and thrift shops can be helpful. If you're really in a creative mood, you can make your own fun containers out of what you already have — shoeboxes, coffee cans, used jars, etc. Ask others to donate their extras too, if you need more. You can paint them, use contact paper, or add other colorful decorations to make them more fun.

What really helped me in the kitchen was getting some clear Lucite containers for jars, bottles, etc., in my fridge, as well as clear glass bowls for washed fruit and veggies. I've been using those for years.

Dividers for drawers are helpful. Even cardboard containers for inside supply cabinets can do wonders. Just think about how to contain things to keep them looking good and organized.

Maintain – Once you finish, check once a month or so to keep order.

You will need to consider if this is the right choice for you based on whether you will be traveling during this time. If you are only gone for a day or two, on those days, you could organize your phone, your emails, your laptop, desktop, or any other digital property.

One more area of organizing that I have just recently discovered is photos. I have tens of thousands of photos on my phone. You probably do too. This has been the hardest thing for me to quickly, pleasantly, and easily solve. Eventually, I did, with an app called ChatBooks that allows you to organize your photos and order a hardback book of the results. There are probably other similar apps, but that is the one I have been using. You can use it on your phone or computer.

I do everything based on the year. I start on the app and choose all of the photos from last year, 2023, and randomly, quickly put them in the app. Then, on my computer, where I can see them larger, I delete the ones that I really don't want. You can put captions on them, too. I did a few, but mostly, I just wanted to accomplish my goal of getting the book done.

That was it, and then I ordered. I received a gorgeous, hardback book of family photos. You can also choose paperback. A few months later, I did the same thing for 2022. Next, I will do 2021, and eventually, I will have a beautiful bookcase with all these books lined up together. Very satisfying!

If You Chose "CREATE" (Or Are Thinking About It)

Did you choose CREATE from BrainWork? This can be a great way to reduce stress. Give yourself a chance to find something that brings you joy. If you engage in this every day, you will likely improve your skill. When you get better at something, it makes you want to do it more.

Maybe you already have a creative hobby or skill you love that reduces your stress and puts you into that flow state where you don't realize how much time has passed. If you never allow yourself time to do it, then this might be for you.

Sometimes, you just have to try something. Read about it. Go to a local store and check out supplies or what you might need. Watch some YouTube videos on the subject. I know a lot of people who want a hobby they enjoy, but they just don't take the time to pursue it. As you prepare for your sixty days, start investigating what you might choose.

Ideas

- Painting (including paint by number)
- Drawing
- Coloring
- Mosaic tile work
- Collage making
- Scrapbooking
- Card making
- Origami
- Needlework (knitting, crochet, sewing, quilting, needlepoint)
- Jewelry making or beading
- Silversmithing
- Creative writing
- Poetry
- Calligraphy
- Pottery
- Sculpting
- Miniature clay art
- Paper mâché
- Soap making
- Basket weaving
- Woodworking
- Glassblowing
- Metalworking
- Gardening
- Flower arranging
- Birdwatching
- Interior design
- Landscape design
- Cooking
- Baking
- Preserving food
- Dance
- Theatre
- Singing
- Learning an instrument
- Songwriting
- Photography
- Bible journaling (there are Bibles with areas on the sides to draw, doodle, create)
- Jigsaw puzzles
- Creating your own flies for fishing (apparently, this is an incredibly creative pursuit. Who knew?)

I have a good friend who is totally into adult coloring books. She puts her finished products out for all to see. She also goes to lots of craft classes and tries other kinds of art, including different forms of painting. She isn't an expert, and most importantly, she isn't afraid to jump in and try.

My friend Gail's favorite pastime is home decorating. She has an eye for color and what looks good together. She has made many of her own curtains and pillows and has even helped me in my house. She loves to change rooms around and decorate for seasons, adding all the little touches.

Find something new that excites you! Everyone is creative; you just have to find an activity that interests you. If you are not sure at all what to do but you want to find something, you could choose exploring hobbies in general for your Sixty-Day Dare. Take those 30 minutes daily to research and try different ideas.

Be Courageous: Exit The Comfort Zone

Remember, we want to be courageous in our choices and in the area of BrainWork. So, pick something that will challenge you. Maybe even something you've been avoiding or resisting.

It takes courage to delve into our background if it is something we have not pursued. It takes courage to make the decision to get into therapy and discuss our most private thoughts with someone. If you choose to do that, get recommendations for a good counselor. You can find them in private practice, through churches, and online.

For some of us, it will take courage to write those Morning Pages out and let whatever is inside come up to the surface. For others, it might take courage to start the process of decluttering and clearing your environment. And if you find you need help, it might take courage to ask someone to help you. However, it can make a huge difference. I have a few friends who are a great help in clearing some of my more difficult areas because they are much more objective than I am.

Trying something new can feel funny and might require courage. If you're meditating, praying, using affirmations, or engaging in a new creative outlet for the first time, you might feel this way.

Remember, you are getting out of your comfort zones here. You are taking a short sixty days to do something new that will make a difference in your life. If you want change, you have to change. You have to set boundaries. You have to set your life up to be successful, and you have to have the courage to do those things.

If not now, then when? Do you want to look back on your life and regret not having had the courage to do the things you wanted to do, or would you rather feel happy about how brave you were and how much fun you had finding all those new things you love to do?

Be Committed: Design Your Fail-Proof BrainWork System

When you've chosen what to do in the BrainWork category, remember to once again look at your calendar and create this part of your plan for your sixty days. If you will be traveling during that time, think through how you will accomplish your goals on travel days. It is absolutely possible, but you will need to plan for it.

You can easily take your writing notebook with you, and you can also take any reading material, podcasts, or audiobooks. You can declutter your digital material if you are on a trip. You can easily meditate and pray. When it comes to Create, think through what you can do to accomplish this daily on a trip. Many hobbies, like needlecrafts or sketching, are small enough to travel with, but others may be more difficult. Get creative and find a solution that will still benefit you.

Remember: Make it SMART

Your goal for the sixty days will need to be something you will do every day, and it will need to be a SMART goal so you can be very clear as to whether or not you accomplished it each day. As a review, a SMART goal is Specific, Measurable, Achievable, Relevant, and Time-Based.

Break it Into Small, Doable Tasks

I have a good friend who, for a long time, wanted to create tile mosaics for garden stepping stones, kitchen trays, and small tabletops. She wanted to make them for herself, as gifts, or even to sell. She was so excited about it for months — but she hadn't started it.

"What the heck are you waiting for?" I asked her one day as we sat in her garden, sipping iced tea.

"I don't know where to begin!" she confessed. "There are so many things to think about. It just seems overwhelming."

"Could you chunk it into different sections?" I asked.

"Maybe," she said, but she was still trying to wrap her brain around it. We kept talking. She got her notebook and started writing down individual "assignments" I was giving her. Doing one small assignment per day makes things much more doable.

The first one was to decide where in her house to set up a workstation. What kind of space did she need? Would she need a special table, a special light, a chair? Storage cabinets for supplies? She needed to gather together the equipment she already had on hand and set it up.

More "assignments" came up. The next was to get the rest of the equipment she needed. Then, she needed to make a list of the supplies she needed for her first project. And then, she needed to buy those — shopping at the hobby store and maybe ordering some things online. Once she got those, she could set up her station.

After that, all she had to do was take a seat and start creating! Breaking it all down like that, into six separate tasks, re-excited her to start the process of creating.

How can you do that same thing? For any large project or goal, how can you divide your preparation into small, doable tasks that are not overwhelming, so you feel comfortable committing to them?

As you're planning, remember your boundaries. Do you need to clear your schedule of anything so you can keep your promises to yourself? Think through how much time you want to give to the choices you have made. Always add in some buffer time because once you're in the moment, you may want to go a little longer than what you planned for. Leave room for that magic!

Write Your BrainWork Goal Down

You've now planned for your BrainWork option. Great job! Now that you've made up your mind, write down your decisions about BrainWork in the same place you wrote your BodyWork choices.

Also, put them on a sticky note and post them, maybe in multiple places, so they start to be in the forefront of your mind as you continue to prepare. The best places for me to post goals are my makeup mirror and my computer. Just somewhere you know you will see daily, if not multiple times a day.

I'm so proud of you!! Let's keep going.

PART FOUR

WORLDWORK

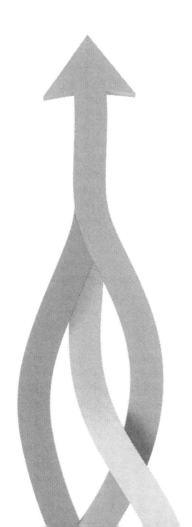

CHAPTER 10

WorldWork – Your Lasting Place in the World

How wonderful it is that nobody need wait a single moment before starting to improve the world.
— ANNE FRANK

Now, we get to turn from an inward focus to an outward focus and enter into WorldWork. This is the super fun and exciting part where you get to do what you were designed by God to do!

If you have already thought about this and are doing it daily, great. However, after decades of giving to others, you may not be at all sure what you should do as you grow older or as you're looking at your broader purpose. You're not alone. I've been there, and most of my friends have too.

WorldWork is a combination of engaging in our purpose, and it's also about our relationships. These two are keys to longevity. Keep in mind that your purpose now could be something you haven't even thought of yet.

Purpose

It is so common for women around our age to start thinking, "It's too late for me to really do something new or make a big difference in the world." Nothing could be further from the truth. I hope by now you know I believe this with all my heart, and I want you to as well!

The world desperately needs you because only you can do what only you can do. I love that thought. I love to think that *I only want to do what only I can do.* That's really all there is time for. There are others who should be doing things that are not meant for me.

Only I can be the wife to my husband the way I do. Only I can mother these particular children the way I do. Only I can write this book the way I write it. Only I can teach a natural health or yoga class like only I can. Maybe I make a difference to someone out there I don't even know, and that difference spurs them on to good things. So those are the things I should spend my precious time doing. And the same goes for you.

We all need you to do what only you can do in the way only you do it. The words you speak, the way you move, the sentences you write, the art you create, the impact you have on one or on thousands. Believe in yourself and gather that courage.

> *We all need you to do what only you can do in the way only you do it.*

Relationships

Northwestern Medicine Psychologist Sheehan Fisher, PhD, tells us the benefits of being in healthy relationships, whether romantic or platonic, include having "... less stress... less production of the stress hormone, cortisol... better healing... healthier behaviors... a greater sense of purpose... [and a] longer life.[78] I don't think any of this is a surprise, and it should certainly be reason enough to get this area right.

Toxic relationships, on the other hand, can be so destructive. Your health, in all ways, suffers. So will your longevity if you don't take action. If you think you are in a toxic relationship, please find a way to get into therapy and understand why and how you got there. You should not be hurt in your relationships, whether physically, mentally, emotionally, sexually, or spiritually. You might have allowed your boundaries to be subtly pushed so far that you don't even realize what has happened.

Our relationships also change, creating stress if we aren't willing to accept that. Our adult children may not want our advice the way we gave it when they were young, and we find it might be best to wait until they ask. Our parents may need us more than they did, and we must find ways to adapt.

If we base our relationship focus on the three keys the researchers found within the healthy centenarian communities, we should follow these tips:

- Put family relationships first.
- Create social circles that nurture us and allow us to nurture others.
- Belong to a faith-based community.

Like anything worthwhile, relationships take work. If we don't take the time to make sure we are tending that "relationship garden," weeds can grow, causing it to deteriorate. Doing the healthy actions listed in BodyWork, BrainWork, and WorldWork categories gives us so much more ability to manage and find great joy in our relationships.

Zone of Genius

Have you ever heard the term "zone of genius?" I love this term. It was coined by Gay Henricks in his book *The Big Leap*. [79]

It's that place or "zone" where each of us is at our best in whatever we are doing in the world. It could be a job, a career, a volunteer situation, an art form — just whatever it is for which we were obviously created.

Forever, I have been fascinated with watching people in their zones of genius. I actually centered my final film project around this basic idea as a senior in college over forty years ago. I created a video with a background of classical music showing five artists going from frustrated and discouraged to being in their flow and creating their beautiful art. There was a writer, a dancer, a violinist, a sculptor, and a painter.

I never really felt like an artist, but I loved the art of creating film and video by bringing all of the artists together to do *their* thing. Oh, yeah, there is a name for that: "producer." That's what I did. I created environments for the artists to shine. Actors, writers, camera people, editors, graphic artists, etc.

I was fascinated with their process and their pursuit, as well as by the exhibition of their art. Such a personal thing. Today, I absolutely love watching the conductor of our local, small-town symphony. I've never seen anyone get so into something. My eyes are always glued on him. You can tell he is in another place, unaware of the audience, when he is conducting.

Purpose is not just about art, though I do think when an engineer is figuring out how something works or when a grandmother is in the midst of a deep, meaningful conversation with a grandchild, each is that person's art.

I want to be in my zone of genius. Don't you? What a great time in your life to pursue it. You will be getting physically healthier as you do the Sixty-Day Dare, and that improvement will help you pursue your dreams. You will be getting mentally healthier, and you need that too. It will help you not worry about things you don't need to worry about and set good boundaries so you can achieve your purpose in the world today.

It is our responsibility to un-apologetically bring our purpose to fruition. That includes you! You are a light in the world. The world needs you.

You are a light in the world. The world needs you.

What is your zone of genius? What gets you into that flow state where you don't know how much time has passed? Don't you love that experience? If you've never had it, don't you want to? Trust me, you do. And once again, it's not too late!

What Your Purpose Does for Others

Once my friend Gail got mentally and physically healthier, she naturally began to put herself out into the world to help others. For a time, she was an activity director at an assisted living residence. She loved it, and the people there loved her.

When those elderly people looked in her face with such thankfulness and gratitude that she was there, listening to them, lifting them up in her special "Gail way," it filled her up. Her emotional tank would, in fact, overflow and allow her to give even more. And when she went home after that, you can bet she was a great partner to her husband because she was filled with that energy and purpose.

Because she is doing what she is really good at, not only is it helping those elderly people, but it is also positively affecting her other relationships. It's like that skipping stone in the water that causes ripples to expand further and further to more and more people.

Maybe she has a conversation with her adult child that night. She is on a high after being deep in her purpose. The conversation is really good and just what that child needs to hear. That child goes on to talk to their spouse, a friend, or a child, and the effects of Gail in her purpose continue to affect more and more people that she doesn't even know about.

Do you see how important this work is to others? Well, now let's look at what it does for you.

How Your Purpose Helps You

Psychology Today reports through a variety of studies that people with purpose "have stronger immune systems, recover more quickly from surgery, and even live longer [which we knew]... have more economic success... [and] are happier.[80]

Those are a lot of good benefits! And, as we can see, they go right along with what the longevity research showed. This is why WorldWork is a category in the Self-Perpetuating Circle of Purpose and a part of the Sixty-Day Dare.

Why People Don't Live Their Purpose

Whether we are helping one specific person continually or thousands of people at a time, when we bring our natural proclivities and abilities together to solve a problem for others, we experience the fulfillment and meaning of life. We help create peace, satisfaction, contentment, and even a legacy.

So why on earth wouldn't we want to do more of this?

It's simple. Doubt comes into our heads. We might think, "Oh, it's too late. By the time I figure it out, no one will want or need this, and there are other people who have already been doing it for 30 years and are experts."

We've already seen that's not true. Stories abound of people doing THEIR thing in the last third of their lives.

Regardless of the truth, we all have that stupid little voice of doubt in our heads. Julia Cameron has written forty books now, and she still has it. She calls it her "censor" and even named him Nigel.

Nigel still rears his nasty head while she writes, saying things like, "This book is a bunch of crap, and no one will want to read it." Julia now just says in her mind, "Oh, it's just you, Nigel. Get lost," and goes back to her work.

If it helps, name that censor and remember who he/she is. We are all in a battle with our minds, and we have to put good things into them for good things to come out.

> We are all in a battle with our minds, and we have to put good things into them for good things to come out.

When you're doubting yourself, remember: Nobody would do it like you! Don't you think God would put people in your life who want to hear YOUR story, in your way, with your twist on things? What if what you say, write, design, or create is just different enough from others' work that it helps someone totally get it when they hadn't before? Wouldn't those people be missing something in their lives without what you have to offer? Yes, for sure!

Don't let that censor win. The most important thing in the world is that we do not end up with regrets at the end of our lives. No regrets allowed. We want to be true to ourselves and our calling, and we want to love the people in our lives well.

Once our time is gone, we cannot get it back. The minutes, the days, the years. How do we make sure we use our precious time on earth in the best way possible? We live it intentionally, not haphazardly. And we do that by living our core values.

Be True to Your Core Values

Understanding your core values is so important in the process of identifying who you are and what you should be doing in the world, and they can change over time. It's important to keep in touch with yourself for that reason.

Do you want to discover your top five core values for this time in your life? I put an exercise in the Sixty-Day Dare DREAM questions for that (see Appendix B).

You can also find lists of core value words online and narrow them down until you come to your top five. Mine are freedom, beauty, truth, intuition, and encouragement. There are many other words that are key for me, but I found that they could fit into one of these five broader categories. I keep them posted at my desk and see them daily.

Knowing the key words that define who you want to be is often helpful in fulfilling your purpose. Post them in your home so you see and remember them, and then form good boundaries that will help them come true.

Once you understand more of who you are and where you came from and have also figured out your core values and the person you desire to be, you can dream. That's pretty exciting!

Dreams that Light Your Fire

Whenever I think of dreams, I think of a recent visit I had with a group of my friends and what happened afterward.

It's late August of the year I turned 60. I'm in Santa Barbara, California in a beautiful rental house high up overlooking the ocean, mountains to the side, and gorgeous hot pink bougainvillea everywhere. I'm hanging out with four wonderful college girlfriends, all of whom also turned 60 this year.

This will be interesting, I think.

As usual, though we are all in a similar stage of life, our situations are all different. Sharon feels retirement is on the horizon. Debra is pondering leaving the job she is in and finding a similar new one. And Jill still has to occasionally deal with her ex (the father of her children) from years ago. Debra is too. Laura is juggling her career, time with her four adult children in various locations, while taking care of her aging parents. I, as usual, am the only one who still has young children at home, and I'm thinking of writing a book.

We gaze out at the Santa Barbara lights, sipping our skinny margaritas and feasting on our dinner of chips, guac, and salsa as we catch up.

"How has your ex been lately?" Jill asks Debra.

"Still such a jerk," Debra replies, scooping a giant heap of guac onto a chip. "I try not to interact with him unless I have to." She pops the chip into her mouth, crunching away.

"That guy at our last college reunion sure seemed interested in you," I point out. "We need to figure out how you two can go on a date!"

Surprised, Debra swallows her chip and takes a giant gulp of her margarita to wash it down. "Oh my gosh, I can't!" she protests as we all laugh. "Dating at this age is brutal."

"How about you? Any cute guys on the horizon?" I ask Jill.

"I'm actually dating someone now," she replies, grinning.

"What?!" we all exclaim, and she starts to laugh now as we immediately bombard her with questions. This interrogation goes on for around ten minutes. When we're satisfied this guy seems like a keeper, we toast him with a clink of our margarita glasses, and then we're on to the next subject.

"Have you heard of that new book, "How Not to Die?" Laura asks us, grabbing a few more chips.

"Really? There's a book with that title?" Sharon says, laughing. She gets up to go find more chips to refill the nearly empty basket on the table.

"Yes, and it's sooooo good!" Laura and I both say. We all get into a heated book discussion, Sharon listening with interest as she does chip refill duty.

The night continues on as we flit from one subject to another — our parents' health, our kids' lives, our spouses, our own health. Around midnight, I ask them the big questions that have been on my mind since turning 60.

"What do you want to do with your life in the next five or ten years?" I ask. "Did you have any dreams when you were younger that you still want to do?"

Things get quieter as everyone starts pondering.

Finally, Jill speaks up. "I've been thinking about that too for the last few years. I'm just not sure, aside from having fun with my kids now that they're grown up and traveling to fun places." Jill was a flight attendant for years. I always thought that was so cool.

"You also sound like you're having fun dating," Sharon points out.

Jill laughs. "Yeah, and that."

"I always wanted to be a fashion designer when I was a kid," Laura says, her eyes lighting up.

"I believe that!" I say. "You have such an ability for dressing so beautifully. I struggle with that. I'd love to see what you'd come up with!"

"I love my job, and it couldn't be better, but I'm getting to the point where they start to encourage retirement," Sharon admits. "I've thought it would be sort of fun to be a health coach of some sort."

"You'd be great at that," Debra tells her. "All our lives, you've prioritized having a healthy body."

"I agree," I say. "When we go on walks, I can barely keep up with you."

We turn to Debra. "I love what I do at my job, but I don't like the culture," she says. "There is too much petty stuff going on. I don't need a new career; I just need a job doing the same thing in a better environment."

We continue talking about these ideas, excited by what each other is saying. No one even notices when all the chips are gone.

Finally, Sharon yawns and looks down at her watch. "Oh my gosh, do you know it's 1:30 a.m.? No wonder I'm tired. Where did the time go?"

We decide to turn in. It's been a beautiful evening, but we do need to sleep. Our weekend together seems to fly by just as quickly, and before we know it, we're hugging each other good-bye with promises to keep in touch.

We weren't able to get together again for a long time, but when we finally did, I got updates on their lives. I so hoped they would be able to do those things they'd talked about or maybe something else that got them excited.

It turns out that Jill married that guy, and they've had a great relationship. Less than a year after their marriage, he was diagnosed with a bad illness, and she became his major caretaker.

"I certainly had no idea this is how things would turn out," she confided one night. "I thought it might overwhelm me, but honestly, our lives have been good, and we don't take a single day for granted." What a deal. She is the true definition of a "helper." Compassionate, sympathetic, warm-hearted. It makes me think God definitely had a plan here.

And Debra did get that new job. "The company is wonderful!" she exclaimed as we met over dinner when we got together. "I love the people, and they really appreciate me. I do the same kind of bookwork, and I also get to head up the welcoming committee."

Sharon is still working full time, but she is looking into the health coaching business as a possible side gig. She's done a ton of research and is already so knowledgeable. Laura has gone to some amazing health conferences in beautiful locations. I'm sure she continues to look stunning everywhere she goes and loves visiting her four adult children who live in far-flung locales. I secretly hope she keeps the fashion design idea on the table!

We all want something to dig into and work on — something that lights our fire, reinvigorates us to press on, and excites us with possibilities every time we think about it. When we pursue THAT thing that makes us feel THAT way, we are absolutely headed in the right direction.

I love the verse, "Take delight in the Lord and He will give you the desires of your heart" (Psalm 37:4, NIV). I take that as some evidence that it is anything but selfish to pursue those dreams. It is what we were made for.

Do you have dreams right now that you can identify that get you excited when you think about them? If not, that first step is to let your mind really wander and not worry about obstacles at the moment. If it's meant to be, the path will open up.

Transforming Trauma

For many people, from trauma comes their purpose in the world or maybe deep insights into how to live. Think back to Gail and her trauma as a child. It actually forced her to pursue therapy and deep understanding of who she is so she could make sense of horrible things and also not let it rule her life in a negative way. She is sensitive, a great listener, and very perceptive. The people she has helped along the way in this second part of her life love her and her caring nature, yet she still has good boundaries so she can make sure she is doing well in all areas of body and brain self-care too.

Recall any trauma you have had. Do you see a path to a new purpose that might have evolved out of the trauma? You may think it didn't allow you to believe you could pursue your purpose, and I certainly understand that. Remember: There is always hope, and we know by now that it is never too late.

When my mother went to therapy after years of struggling with *her* childhood trauma, her therapist said something I'll never forget. "It's time to walk out of that tomb and into the light. You've been there long enough." That made her feel so much better.

Self-Reflection: Where Are You with WorldWork?

Have you been working on a strong purpose that excites you and reignites your passion for life that will take you through the next five to ten years? If so, what is it? Are you focused on continuing it, or do you feel you need to change something?

Are you clear on your current core values? Are you manifesting them in the things you do?

How are your relationships? Do you have a few friends and family whom you can count on, and who can count on you? If not, why?

Do you pursue spiritual or religious gatherings and discussions? Are they helping you fulfill your purpose and build supportive relationships?

Have you felt a longing to do something more or different in the world?

What would you do now for the next five to ten years if there were absolutely no obstacles? Could you take some baby steps to check into that? Could you research something? Look into an online course? Read a book or ask someone some questions?

Keep these things in mind as we look at the WorldWork Big Five.

CHAPTER 11

The WorldWork Big Five: Rotate and Balance

If you can dream it, you can do it.
— **WALT DISNEY**

The WorldWork Big Five are a little different from the previous Big Five in that you don't necessarily just pick one. You can either choose:

- **DREAM** – Write the answer to one Dream Question a day. (See Appendix B for the 60 DREAM Questions.)

Or you can rotate among any or all of the WorldWork Big Five options. (See "How It Works" further down in this chapter for more details.) The rest of the Big Five are:

- **ENGAGE** – Have a positive, intentional connection with family, friends, or other relationships. This means a conversation back and forth — on the phone, in person, or on video chat. More than just a text.
- **GATHER** – Go to something spiritual, such as a gathering, event, small group, intimate get-together, book club, church, one-on-one meeting, etc.
- **HELP** – Volunteer to help anyone with anything and enjoy yourself.
- **ACT** – Spend an hour or more on your mission, vision, or purpose if you know what it is or are trying on something new for size.

Since you can choose to rotate among these, it will be important to have your Sunday Planning session each week (see this process in Chapter 13) to plan your week.

Why These Five?

It's time to generate the fullness of life we all want. I picked these Big Five because they are central to all of our longevity studies and are also basic common sense in terms of what we do in the world — our purpose and relationships.

Once again, we are going from that inward focus of getting our bodies and minds healthy to accomplish the outward focus of our place in the world. What did God design us to do and with whom did He want us to be in relationship? These are, most definitely, the things we will care about at the end of our lives.

Who Do You Want to Be?

The line, "Decide who I want to be," is from one of my favorite books, *Atomic Habits* by James Clear.[81]

When I first heard that line, I thought it was ridiculous. Decide who I want to be? I am who I am, aren't I? Well, yes, and that is also part of the problem.

The messages we got as children have etched deep grooves into our subconscious. Unless we have done a lot of self-development work — therapy, journaling etc. — those messages may still be running us today. If they are running us in a wonderful, positive way, that is awesome! However, there could be areas that are not serving us well in the arena of digging into a new direction and/or sharing our gifts with the world.

This is why that BrainWork is so important to your WorldWork. You know if you have things to work through. If so, do it and get started on your WorldWork too.

Having lived as long as we both have, I know you have some wisdom that someone, maybe more than one, needs.

#1: DREAM – Guidelines and Ideas

If you don't yet have a clear vision of your path, take time to dream about what your purpose or your future could be.

You know the old saying: "Where there is no vision, the people perish" (Proverbs 29:18, KJV).

Your dream is your destination, and your goals are the steps along the way. Having a clear dream or purpose makes it easier to stay focused and committed. A future purpose you can sink your teeth into can be difficult to identify, so do not feel bad about not having it figured out. You can definitely get there!

One thing I always loved back in my homeschooling years that I got from the Charlotte Mason homeschool theories was that, very often, kids need time to just sit and dream and be with their thoughts. Their schedules shouldn't be so busy that this doesn't happen. Well, the same goes for us right now. Take that time!

As Brian and Gabrielle Bosché say in their book *The Purpose Factor*,[82] our purpose emanates from our natural advantage or what comes second nature to us, our acquired skills, the problem we like to solve in the world around us, and our moment or series of moments that most shaped our perspective.

Do you have any ideas you could pursue today that would be steps toward a dream you have? If not, that's ok. This is the area where you will begin your exploration into your purpose.

If you do have an idea that keeps sticking around in your brain, think about how Elizabeth Gilbert describes the creative process in her book *Big Magic: Creative Living Beyond Fear*.[83]

According to Gilbert, an idea has a life of its own and zooms around all over the world, finally coming to light on a person who could bring that idea to life in some creative form. If that person agrees to do it — agrees to this partnership — then the idea is born. If not, it will leave after a time to find another willing person to bring it to life.

We do have to jump on those ideas when they come if life permits. I sort of think about this book in that way. The idea came to me on that July 4th morning. I'd been searching for months for that next thing I could get excited about and really dive into. I knew I had to jump on it, and Gilbert's comments sure solidified that idea! I highly recommend her book.

It was after those seven months of delving into my life that the significant experiences, both high and low, my natural gifts, skills learned, and personality traits all collided into a new purpose. That is what the sixty days of DREAM questions can do for you if you choose them as your WorldWork option.

You will need patience. You will need to leave room for the magic to happen (remember boundaries), and you will also need to learn to relax, de-stress, and listen to that still, small voice pointing you in the right direction. With intention, belief, and prayer, your purpose will be revealed for the next part of your life. (See Appendix B for the 60 DREAM Questions.)

#2: ENGAGE – Guidelines and Ideas

"Loneliness is a prevalent and global problem for adult populations, and a number of different studies have linked it to multiple chronic conditions..." says a Pub Med study.[84]

So many things are changing as you get to mid-life and beyond. Reduced roles due to retirement, children leaving the home as adults, the death or illness of a partner, diminished health, losing friends or family. All of these contribute to more loneliness, less connection, and fewer relationships.

The studies show us that relationships impact our emotional health and our physical health; hence, we see this as a major contributor to longevity. They give us feelings of connection, companionship, support, and purpose. We are able to get through tough times better. Bottom line: we were created to be in relationship.

The ENGAGE option will have you intentionally engage with another person in conversation or connection of some sort. It should be positive, loving, non-judgmental, and moving a needle forward in your relationship with that person.

For this category, you might want to engage with your children, your spouse, your friends or acquaintances, or even the guy who bags your groceries at the store. You might want to invite someone for coffee. You might want to do a video call with an out-of-town relationship.

If you are more of an introvert or you just don't have too many people to talk to, you might choose to go to an event. A church is always a welcoming place to start to make yourself have a conversation with someone. The person sitting next to you, the greeter at the door, or anyone you see sitting by themselves. Compliment them. Be curious. Ask them questions about themselves. People love that.

I'm sure the people at a retirement home would be happy to have a visitor. This is simply a habit we need to cultivate within ourselves. If you want good friendships, you must be a good friend.

#3: GATHER – Guidelines and Ideas

In all Blue Zones regions, centenarians were part of religious communities. Dan Buettner, explorer and author of *Blue Zones*, says:

> *A recent study in the* Journal of Health and Social Behavior *followed 3,617 people for seven and a half years and found that those who attended religious services at least once a month reduced their risk of death by about a third... The NIH-funded Adventist Health Study had similar findings. It followed more than 34,000 people over a period of twelve years and found that those who went to church services frequently were 20 percent less likely to die at any age.*
>
> *It appears that people who pay attention to their spiritual side have lower rates of cardiovascular disease, depression, stress, and suicide, and their immune systems seem to work better... To a certain extent, adherence to a religion allows them to relinquish the stresses of everyday life to a higher power.*[85]

This choice specifically pertains to gathering in a small or large group for the purpose of deepening your spiritual connection with each other and a higher power.

According to the Pew Research Center, "83 percent of all U.S. adults believe people have a soul or spirit in addition to their physical body."[86] This is a good reason for most people to believe attending to that part of our lives would be important.

For some, this is already part of your life and won't be too difficult. For others, this is not something you do on a regular basis. You will need to seek out some options for yourself. Ideally, you would do this in person, but if that isn't possible, then online is an option. There are online groups for absolutely every subject under the sun. You can search online for a video call group for a meeting of this type where you will be able to interact.

Churches and other centers of spiritual growth usually meet weekly. In addition, there are often small group meetings at these places, and almost always, some are for women only. I just started a women's Bible study this summer on the subject of untangling emotions. I'm an introvert and can easily just stay home, but stepping out and attending these kinds of groups has always been wonderful for studying and being around welcoming people.

There have been many times in my life when I have met weekly with a few female friends, usually about three to six, for about two hours to talk about our lives and then write down in a journal what each person needed prayer for that week. During our week, we would pray about those things for each person.

We also, typically, wanted accountability for something. So, we would tell each other the thing we wanted to do, and we would all write it down in our pretty journals, and then we would report back the next week. This kind of group can be a lifeline. Every woman I've ever discussed this with has said how necessary it was for her emotional and mental health. I think it goes back thousands of years. Women need to gather and talk and confide and gain strength from other women.

You could also meet with one person for spiritual guidance. There are Christian counselors, spiritual counselors, church pastors, and just other people who are simply well-versed in what you are looking for. Meeting one-on-one would satisfy this "gathering" category to learn, explore, discuss, and up-level your life in this area.

The goal of all of this is to encourage each other. We all need it. Life can be a struggle, and this is how we strengthen each other in the journey.

#4: HELP – Guidelines and Ideas

The health benefits of volunteering have been well studied and documented. It can get you out of the anxiety of focusing on your own problems and, instead, feel useful helping someone in need. You can meet new people and even develop a support system through it. Many find their purpose through it. Do a little research on all the health benefits of volunteering.

For these reasons, the HELP choice is all about volunteering. It's easy to feel busy and not have time for this, but it doesn't have to cost a lot of time, and the benefits can be huge. Of course, this also falls into the category of relationships, even though you might volunteer to help someone do something without them knowing it.

You could make this as simple as rolling your neighbor's trash can back up to its spot after the garbage truck comes. Or, you could participate in places that feed the hungry, help counsel teen moms, take meals to the homebound, help your adult children with their children, work with animals, or work in a community garden.

Another option is to be on a board or help with various local government departments or non-profit organizations. Or maybe work on a political campaign. They always need volunteer citizens to get involved. Check out what might be near you.

Do an online search for all of the different ways a person can volunteer and I'm sure you can find something that will help someone else that also interests you. This is about taking the focus off of yourself and putting it on someone else. Sometimes, making the effort to do this immediately gives you a new view on your life. It is meaningful and fulfilling, and it could lead to a new purpose.

I remember one of my favorites was being a "baby holder" at the public hospital in downtown Los Angeles. I was single and in my thirties. The babies had been born to mothers on drugs. The mothers had been arrested, and the babies were in withdrawal. It was very intense. I just sat in a rocking chair, rocked the babies, and did whatever the nurses instructed. It was one of the best volunteer jobs I've ever had.

#5: ACT – Guidelines and Ideas

Creating a habit of attending to your purpose or your mission on a daily basis is what will get you to your ultimate goal. To write this book, I had to devote daily time to writing. Otherwise, it never would have come to fruition.

This choice is for the person who knows their purpose or has an idea they want to explore as a purpose. It is to work for at least an hour a day with focused attention on that thing. If you can determine your most productive hours of the day, it would be ideal to do your work during that time. If not, it's no big deal.

Here are some examples of what purpose could look like:

- Make a difference in politics on a topic you are passionate about by getting involved.
- Educate people on the history of your local town by writing a book.
- Create a side business, whether online or brick-and-mortar, to help people dress better to fit their body type.
- Increase your income by renovating a house and flipping it or getting into real estate or Airbnb.
- Take care of your grandkids a certain amount of time per week and purpose to teach them good things so they grow up to be good citizens of the world.
- Learn a new skill or get certified in something so you can help others in those areas.
- Challenge yourself physically, possibly with a sport and cooking super healthy, and then help others do the same.

If you're not sure, go back to the DREAM section.

You will need to plan where this work will take place. Do you need to rearrange your life to be able to have that focus without interruption? Will this affect other people, and do you need to discuss it with them?

If you really want to dedicate yourself to making strides in this area, you could choose to do this every day for the sixty days or at least most of the days and choose something else for some breaks along the way.

You'll understand more about that when you see "How it Works" below.

Maybe your purpose is teaching art to kids or participating in a local theater group or something that doesn't take place at your home. You might have some of your experiences in that location, and you also might need to do prep work at home or, again, somewhere else. The point is to schedule dedicated time for this.

Wherever you are working, create a distraction-free environment. Turn off digital notifications and organize your workspace to be attractive to you. Make sure you have a good chair if you are sitting, good lighting, and good temperature. I have a little white mini fan on my desk in case I get a hot flash, usually after drinking a hot drink, so I can just keep writing on through it.

Set those boundaries for yourself and others. Maybe you need a little sign on your door that says, "Please do not disturb." Maybe turn off your phone and log out of your social accounts for a certain time period. You can schedule a time when you are not at your prime creative self or in serious production mode to read emails, go through social accounts, or return texts and calls. Don't do those things during your best creative time of day.

You can also use something called the Pomodoro. Basically, it is working completely focused on your task for 25 minutes, then taking a five-minute break. Stretch, walk around, get a drink or snack, or go to the bathroom. Then, back for another 25 minutes. This is good for groups working on a project too. You get focused bursts, maximum productivity, and time efficiency.

If you feel you need more support on this, I've even been on video calls called a "Power Hour," where we all were focused on our own tasks at our desks, and one person was the timer. We would do fifteen-minute focused work, and then we could stay on that or move to a different task every quarter hour. There was no talking. Just the leader. You are there with all these other people working on their tasks. Everyone is in the same boat. It's pretty cool!

For some, it is mostly about dedicating time, setting goals, and getting tasks done. For others, it is about gathering courage and taking steps that might be scary at first. For still others, it is about saying no to some things that are taking up your time, but when you think about it, they really don't fit into the vision of the life you desire. Saying no can be hard, but if you don't say no, your vision won't happen, and you'll end up with regret. This happens too often.

How It Works

Unlike the BodyWork and BrainWork sections, in WorldWork you have two options for how to proceed.

Option 1: DREAM Focus – If you are unsure of your current purpose, I recommend you focus only on the DREAM segment and answer one question a day for 60 days. Even if you know your purpose and you are already working on it, you can still choose this option. It is a good idea to revisit your answers to these questions periodically. Every few years, things can definitely change.

Option 2: Big Five Rotation – Our second option in WorldWork is to rotate among any or all of the Big Five. Each day, choose to do at least one thing in any of the categories. This is a good way to find that balance we want in our lives. Cogitate on what you need most.

Starting Smart: Shift Your Mindset

I know that by engaging in some of the Big Five WorldWork options, you might really be pushed out of your comfort zone — or you might feel really excited. Or maybe a little of both. Either way, just think what can happen in sixty days.

Small, incremental improvements lead to a changed life — in this case, a life of meaning and fulfillment and being able to get to the end with great satisfaction and contentment. I don't care if you are far away from anything we are talking about in this book. There is a starting place for you, and you CAN take baby steps.

Have you decided which of the Big Five in WorldWork speak to you the most? Are you thinking more about purpose or more about various relationships, or is it all of the above?

The great thing about this section is the ability to rotate among the options. It's not my favorite thing to tell someone, "You should do this or that," but honestly, with our goal being longevity and health and happiness and good things, these are the proven facts so, yes, if we want a life well-lived, we "should" all be doing all of them, in one capacity or another.

If something turns you off, could you possibly dip your toe in and just try it? You've heard me say it before: If we want change in our lives, we must change what we have been doing. I know you've probably heard that definition of insanity: Doing the same thing over and over again, expecting a different result. So, let's change things up. You'll never know till you try!

Commit: Write Down Your WorldWork Choice

I so wish I could talk to you right now and ask you what you are thinking. How are you feeling? You've moved through BodyWork, BrainWork, and now WorldWork. Good job, my friend!

It's time to write down now what you want to focus on in WorldWork. Put it with the others, and let's go on to start thinking about some ways to make it work for you. We're in the home stretch now!

CHAPTER 12

Planning Your WorldWork

Vision without action is merely a dream.
Action without vision just passes the time.
Vision with action can change the world.
— JOEL A. BARKER

SMART and Balanced

Take a moment and look at what you've chosen in each of the three categories. BodyWork, BrainWork, and WorldWork. If you still aren't quite sure, write out the choices you're trying to decide between and then write out the details that make them SMART goals. Specific, Measurable, Achievable, Relevant, and Time-Based.

Think about how your days will go when you add these new items to your schedule. Do you need to cancel or take a break from certain other activities for these sixty days? Think that through. Write out some sample days. A weekday. A weekend. This will set you up to win.

The Focus Is Now on You

Everything you did in the last twenty to thirty years has been so important. No doubt about it. You are or were the hub of your family. It all revolved around you, didn't it? Maybe it still does. If you're a mama, raising and molding those little human beings is the most important thing you've ever done. Good job! Even if things aren't the way you planned them, I know you did the best you could at the time. Don't we all?

However, in this book, we are talking about YOU today: *your* health and *your* dreams.

Not your children.

Not your spouse.

Not your previous work.

Just you.

Right? Let's figure out how to make all of this work together — for YOU. Because if you get your own oxygen mask on, you'll be even better at doing what you do best — helping others in only the way you can do it.

Be Curious

Watch for Signs

For a while, my WorldWork was adopting two children from foreign countries. This WorldWork and spiritual BrainWork came together one day when I was having serious doubts.

We had brought our fourth child home from Russia a couple of years prior. We were in the midst of the paperwork to bring our fifth child home from Ethiopia, and I was one month away from turning fifty.

Here we go again with the decade birthdays. *Oh, my goodness, what in the holy name of all that is good am I doing? Am I too old to bring a new baby home? Am I crazy?* I was having serious doubts about the rationality of it all.

I was sitting at my table and pulled my Bible over. I said, "Lord, I need you to speak to me somehow, some way, and let me know if I'm really doing the right thing." I decided to just open the book to a random page and hope something there would give me a sign.

Well, it was pretty shocking to see what was on those two pages.

On the left side, I had opened to John 8:57 (NIV). Believe it or not, this verse said, "You are not yet fifty years old." Are you kidding me? I don't even care what the context here is. It actually says that? *Uhhhh... okay, Lord. You definitely have my attention.*

I kept reading. On the right side of the page, starting at John 10:14 (NIV), it said, "I am the good shepherd; I know my sheep and my sheep know me — just as the Father knows me and I know the Father — and I lay down my life for the sheep. I have other sheep that are not of this sheep pen. I must bring them also. They too will listen to my voice, and there shall be one flock and one shepherd."

Good gracious, I still have to get that last sheep into my flock, I thought. From then on, my doubts were quelled.

I believe God gives us what we need in whatever way we can receive it. Some of us need it more tangibly than others.

My main point here is to be alert and curious when the signs come. Ask, and you may get answers in ways you do not expect. Knock, and doors will open to you. We must take action, and we must listen to our gut, our intuition — that still, small voice. Remember, no regrets. Ask God to open your eyes to the signs along the way and also to reveal the best plan for you.

Be Creative: How Can You Make It Fun/Efficient?

How can you create your entire Sixty-Day Dare in a way that makes it doable for you? Well, of course, everyone is in a different situation, and one idea will work for some, but not for others.

The point here is to design a plan that you want to do. Be creative in planning how you can batch things together and how you can set up your environment to trigger your desired behavior.

A Few Examples

If you are going to engage in these sixty days, then play hard. Whatever that means for you. Make it count.

If you are going to engage in these sixty days, then play hard. Whatever that means for you. Make it count.

1. For the hard-core person who knows their purpose and is just now digging into it:

BodyWork: If you are the hard-core type, I'm betting you have already gotten pretty decent at some of the options in this section. I would tell you to choose what seems most difficult for you at this time. Maybe it's a stricter, clean diet with a protein focus and no alcohol or sugar (as in desserts). Maybe it's a harder or longer daily workout.

BrainWork: Perhaps you take the time to sit and read 10 pages a day of a self-improvement book and finish the book before you go on to another. I LOVED doing that in 75 Hard.

You also might want to choose CREATE if you haven't taken the time for that kind of thing in your life.

WorldWork: Remember, you can rotate these, but if you feel you need to dig into working on your purpose, choose ACT and devote an hour a day for five days a week.

One day a week, you could choose ENGAGE and have that intentional, purposeful conversation with someone close to you that you feel you need to encourage or develop.

And on the 7th day of the week, choose GATHER and work on that spiritual component.

Think about batching certain items together. I actually like to work on my purpose right after I work out. My brain is energized at that time.

2. For more of a middle ground and also maybe for someone who is dealing with lots of stress:

BodyWork: Of course, almost everything we have talked about addresses stress, but some may appeal to you more than others. You might start with the MOVE option, or maybe the BREATHE option. If you're like me, BREATHE will be easy to do when you wake up, so you might put a sticky note on your bedside table to remind you in the morning.

BrainWork: If stress is big, you may want to do those Morning Pages and WRITE to get what's in your head out. Alternatively, you could choose BREATHE or MEDITATE. Once you establish a deep breathing pattern, you might be able to do them all at the same time. Try it and see. The CREATE option might also be an enjoyable de-stressor.

WorldWork: If you are under high stress, I'm guessing it might be time for you to **take** time to DREAM and answer those sixty questions in writing. One question per day. You could easily combine this time with writing your Morning Pages if you choose that. Think about batching things together if possible.

3. For the overwhelmed person who needs a simple, easy way to start without a lot of planning:

BodyWork: Of course, this depends on which one you know you need the most. If it is EAT, choose one food item to eliminate from your diet or add one new supplement. If you know you don't drink enough water, DRINK ½ your body weight in ounces of water per day. If you know you need exercise, choose MOVE. Just go for a daily walk. Easy! If you can do 30-45 minutes, that would be ideal. These choices would all be quite simple if you chose just one.

BrainWork: If you choose to walk for BodyWork, it would be easy to add headphones and listen to anything self-improvement oriented, whether personal or business-related (READ), or you could pray or do affirmations during that time too (MEDITATE).

You could record those affirmations on your phone and listen to them while you walk. That's a pretty cool thing to do. Depending on the state of your home, though, CLEAR might be important for you too. If you've got your own version of my cluttered bookcase, let's get to organizing!

WorldWork: I would definitely choose DREAM for you. It is easy to just answer one question a day for the sixty days, and if you are in overwhelm mode, this quiet time for reflection may be exactly what you need to sort out what you want your future to look like. You would just need to determine what time of day you would do it.

4. For The Beginner:

BodyWork: I think MOVE is the best way to start. This can be as little as you need it to be just to get that ball rolling. It can be five-minutes or a walk to the end of the block and back. You decide. If that seems too difficult, choose DRINK so you get that all-important water in.

BrainWork: I'm leaning toward READ here, with particular focus on educating yourself about natural health and longevity.

Remember, you can also listen to a podcast or audiobook on these subjects. Choose one podcast a day or a certain amount of time with an audiobook while doing other things, like puttering around the house or walking or gardening or cleaning out your closet. There are so many good books out there.

WorldWork: You can rotate through these depending on what is speaking to you, but I am definitely leaning toward ENGAGE so you can be in relationships with people that will encourage you. Also GATHER so again, your spirit can be nourished by others. Of course, the DREAM option would probably be a great choice too.

Each day, you could alternate among these three. DREAM (answer one question per day – you don't have to get through all sixty this time around), then ENGAGE, then GATHER.

Design the plan that will work for you.

Design the plan that will work for you.

Be Courageous: Challenge Yourself

Again, I want to emphasize that you make sure to challenge yourself in each of the three categories, but not so much that it will become demotivating. Don't choose things you are already doing on a regular basis unless you want to increase what you are doing. Use these sixty days to make a real difference in your life.

For instance, when I did 75 Hard, I was already doing a 40-minute Pilates class three to five days a week. I really thought hard about whether I could also add 45-minute walk seven days a week, plus 45 minutes of yoga (stretching) on Saturdays and Sundays.

I mean, how hard is it to just walk? I didn't have to go fast. I could meander if I wanted. And worst case, on the weekend, I could literally just sit on my yoga mat and stretch. It was really just a matter of setting aside the time to do it.

Think about your situation. What can you add that is doable, yet may just require you to devote more time to it?

Be Committed: Design a Fail-Proof System

Let's look at some ways you can design the perfect system for your life. It will involve prepping, scheduling your day, and a discussion of habits.

Time to Prep

Here is a list of items you may want to consider depending on your Sixty-Day Dare choices:

- Reorganize my refrigerator, putting my fruit and veggies in clear containers at eye level so that I see them first.
- Find that pretty journal my friend gave me last year to use for my writing, affirmations, and prayers.
- Pull out that old paint-by-numbers kit I got two years ago and set it up in the corner by the window with a good chair and lamp.
- Find or acquire two 32-ounce water bottles so I can have them ready every day.
- Figure out what I'm going to wear to exercise in and set my tennis shoes out in a spot where I see them every day.
- Prep my bedroom for good sleep.
- Make a list of books I want to read and make sure I have them — either order them or get them from the library.
- Get nice containers to help me organize my home so it isn't so cluttered.
- Purchase healthier products so I have a toxin-free home.
- Order some supplements and oils so they are here when my Sixty-Day Dare starts.
- Set up my special spot to read, write, meditate, pray, dream.
- Make a list of people I want to engage with and develop those relationships more.
- Do some research to figure out where I want to gather in a spiritual setting. Also, find out when some women's groups are meeting.
- Look into volunteer opportunities near me.
- Decide what I need to do to get ready to work on my purpose daily. What phone calls do I need to make? Who should I text? Set up my desk better and more

inviting. Do some research online. Make a list of ten-minute tasks and then start to go through them.

Scheduling Your Day

Where can you add your new plans into your day? Remember to also give yourself a little extra buffer time around these as you get used to this new way of living.

You might need extra time to prep your water bottles or prep your food each day or each weekend if you do food prep like that.

You'll need to add in the time devoted to reading, writing, creating, helping, or gathering.

Some days, there are fewer things, but on the days when there is a lot going on, you may need to write out when you will take a bath, do makeup, and get dressed, or when you will work on a project.

A Combo Calendar: Best for Both Worlds

For me, what really works is a combination of my phone calendar and a paper calendar. My phone is always with me, so that is where everything goes first.

My paper calendar/planner has a month and week view, plus an area for notes for that week and that month. This lives where I sit for my morning routine. Transferring things to the paper calendar for each month and week every now and then helps me see the big picture and whether I am cramming too much into certain areas. Along with my big yearly calendar on the wall, these make me feel organized and that, hopefully, I am managing things pretty well.

Your goal is good, new habits, so you need to understand a little science of habits.

Habits and Staying the Course

We've all heard the terrible stats of how most people quit their New Year's resolutions shortly after beginning. The gyms are busy in January but thin out right after that first month of the year. How do we make sure we complete what we set out to do?

Basically, we follow this book. We have a deep desire to make changes in specific areas, and we create goals. We make them SMART goals. We write them down in multiple places, so we see them often. We prepare our environments to be successful. We find a way to be accountable, whether with friends or some sort of program. Hopefully, these goals will become new habits.

These are the basics. Employ what we are discussing in this book, and you should find success.

You could also join our Sixty-Day Dare program (see the back of the book for details).

We unconsciously engage in habits. In *Atomic Habits*[87], James Clear writes about the science of how habits work:

"First, there is a cue. The cue triggers your brain to initiate a behavior."

Maybe you see cupcakes on a table and grab one or you see someone doing something and so you do it too, or maybe you are bored or depressed, and that cues you to eat ice cream or binge-watch TV. Clear continues:

Cravings are the second step, and they are the motivational force behind every habit. ... What you crave is not the habit itself, but the change in state it delivers. You do not crave smoking a cigarette, you crave the feeling of relief it provides. You are not motivated by brushing your teeth but rather by the feeling of a clean mouth.

The third step is the response. The response is the actual habit you perform, which can take the form of a thought or an action. ... Finally, the response delivers a reward. Rewards are the end goal of every habit. The cue is about noticing the reward. The craving is about wanting the reward. The response is about obtaining the reward.

Remember what Clear said earlier about how to build better habits. "Make it obvious [Lay out your tennis shoes]... Make it attractive [Find some cute exercise clothing]... Make it easy [Just head out the door and go walk]... Make it satisfying [Listen to a podcast or walk with a friend, and you'll feel better after you do it]." Considering those four keys can help as we design our Sixty-Day Dare.

Environment Triggers Behavior

I've mentioned this a lot, I know, but it will help us the **most** in the formation of these new habits for a healthier lifestyle.

Environment triggers behavior.

These three words have become a mantra for me. My friends will tell you that I say them all the time.

Clear agrees that the environment is the most powerful trigger. He says, "Motivation is overrated. Environment often matters more." If the priority is optimal health, then setting up one's environment to be successful is key and critical. If you don't do this step first, the results will show. This is also key in the Blue Zones. Their environments nudge them to be more active, to be in more relationships, etc.

Clear also notes that humans have around 11 million sensory receptors in their bodies, 10 million of which are for sight. "Some experts estimate that half of the brain's resources are used on vision," he wrote. It's therefore not surprising that visual cues make a huge difference in our behavior. "A small change in what you see can lead to a big shift in what you do," he wrote. "Imagine how important it is to live and work in environments filled with productive cues and devoid of unproductive ones." [88]

Let's read a bit more of what Dr. Caroline Leaf says about habits and, according to science, how long they take to create.

Leaf states in her book, *Switch on Your Brain*, that it does not take 21 or 30 days, as many have said, to create a new habit. It takes two to eight months, depending on the habit, because you have to create long-term memory, and this takes time. We can actually see the formation take place.

Leaf explains how we can literally see this process of memory imprinting happening in the brain on the dendritic spines of the nerve cells, which form part of the synapse. They change shape by deposited phosphate groups — from a bump to a lollipop, and eventually to a mushroom shape. As long-term memory is fully established in our brains, our thoughts become automatized into habits. [89]

Reassess: Has Your Decision Changed?

What are you thinking, girlfriend? Have you changed your mind at all as you have read through these last few chapters? Are your choices lined out?

I hope you are excited about this. I really believe this is the beginning of a new part of your life.

Ready to finalize your plans? Let's do that next.

PART FIVE

PUTTING THE PLAN TOGETHER

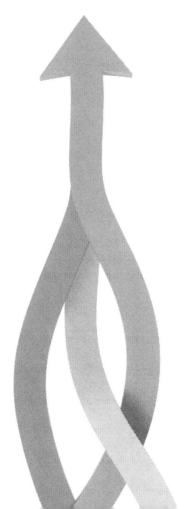

CHAPTER 13

Finalize Your Framework

People with clear, written goals accomplish far more in a shorter period of time than people without them could ever imagine.
— BRIAN TRACY

We've gone through a lot of information and thinking in this book, and I hope you've learned something that you feel is helpful. It's time to pull everything together with some final tips, but first let's talk about Bonnie.

Before & After

Bonnie is a typical woman of about 58 years old. She has been married for 25 years and has three kids, ages 23, 21, and 18. Let's compare her life before and after she improved her habits.

BEFORE

Bonnie rolls out of bed, rushes to get a cup of coffee, then showers, dresses, and jumps in the car to get to work. She hasn't had any water to drink yet today. She arrives at work just in the nick of time. She drinks coffee all morning to have the energy to do the job. At around 10:00 a.m., she grabs a donut from the kitchen.

She drinks a lot of liquids — sodas, tea, coffee, juice — all day, so she doesn't feel thirsty.

When it gets near lunchtime, Bonnie doesn't know what she will eat. Like most days, she assumes she'll probably work through lunch, snacking on vending-machine food instead of eating a full meal. However, her co-workers ask her to go to lunch with them today. At the restaurant, she gets a hamburger, fries, a soda, and a chocolate shake.

Back at the office, she drinks more coffee and another caffeinated soda to make it through that afternoon slump, though she definitely has the jitters from the caffeine and sugar she's consumed. She is depleted and hyped up at the same time. Walking past the kitchen mid-afternoon, she sees a plate of cookies someone has put on the table and grabs a few for a snack. Maybe that will pep her up.

Bonnie is pretty stressed out in general. She misses her kids. They seem to only text her when they need something, not to really talk. They are all young adults now, and figuring out how to communicate with them is a whole new thing. The thought of it brings a heavy sigh.

She also doesn't like her job. She'd really like to quit and try something different, but she thinks it's probably too late in her life or career to change course.

It seems like nobody appreciates her. She struggles with some depression. Today is no different, and she can't wait for the workday to be finished.

By 5:00 p.m., she is exhausted. She drives home and flops on the couch. Bonnie doesn't think much about exercise. It's too hard, and she is too tired. She doesn't think a short walk will make much difference, and she has other important things to do anyway. She is gaining more and more weight, and on top of that, these hot flashes are just too much.

Bonnie's husband wants her to go on a walk with him in the evening, but she doesn't have the energy. At the same time, she sees more and more distance between them but can't seem to do anything about it.

Eventually, she gets up, checks the fridge, and decides on a frozen pizza and some TV because, well, she deserves it. She worked hard today. She ends up having a glass of wine and a prescription sleeping pill to get to sleep.

Despite the pill, Bonnie still doesn't sleep well. She wakes up with night sweats in the middle of the night and is too uncomfortable to get back to sleep for a while. When she does, she breathes through her mouth and snores, waking herself back up. She wonders if she needs to go to a doctor again. She tosses and turns all night, then gets up the next day and does it all again.

AFTER

It took Bonnie some time to get to this point, and she took baby steps in all the areas. However, this is her life now.

Bonnie gets up an hour earlier than she used to and gives herself some time to wake up. She does some deep breathing exercises before getting out of bed. This takes about 10 minutes and allows her time to clear her mind and do a little mediation and prayer too.

As she sits on the edge of her bed, she drinks quite a bit of water from the water bottle she had on her nightstand from the night before. She knows she gets dehydrated overnight. She's a lot better at noticing when she's dehydrated now that she is drinking more water.

Seeing her tennis shoes where she purposely left them the night before, she is triggered to put on her walking clothes first thing. She still gets a cup of coffee, but it's from a brand her research has shown is actually good for her. Taking her water with her, she goes to her special chair, which she has set up as a morning writing station. She has her new journal to write in, her colored pens, and the book she is reading, as well as a table to put her water bottle on. This is her favorite chair, and she loves the view from this spot. She takes some time to download what's in her brain into her notebook and make a plan for the day and the week. After that, she reads ten pages from her book. She's almost finished with it, which is exciting because it's the second one this month. She didn't use to finish many books.

Her essential oils are sitting there, too, as another reminder. She puts several drops of one on her thyroid to help that area, another on her adrenals for good energy, another on her abdomen for hormonal balance, and a fourth on her liver area to keep that healthy. Then, she inhales deeply with each one from her cupped hands. The oil molecules will help her brain, emotions, and memory.

She heads outside with her husband for a thirty-minute morning walk, as they do on most days. This is the time they get their best talks in. She is thankful for that and feels closer to him than she used to. She also gets that wonderful early-morning light in her eyes that helps her circadian rhythm and all the good, brain-happy hormones like dopamine and serotonin that give her a sense of well-being. She feels great.

She gets back and takes a quick shower, using toxin-free shampoo and soap, puts on her toxin-free makeup, gets dressed, and grabs the containers of food she prepped the evening before. This time, they contain fruit and a hard-boiled egg for the morning when she gets to work, and for lunch, she'll have tuna salad and veggies. She's also packed an afternoon snack of plain yogurt, fruit, and some homemade granola.

She grabs one of the little baggies of supplements she prepped at the beginning of the month to take to work each day. She'll take these with breakfast. Some are for hormone balance, some are for joint health, and there are others, too. Between these and the essential oils, her hormone symptoms have definitely subsided. She gets a hormone saliva test done yearly now through her naturopath doc, and the results are good! She heads to work feeling balanced and healthy.

While on a break at work, she dedicates 10 minutes to clearing out the digital clutter on her phone. Then, she sends a text to her brother to see if they can arrange a video call for one night this week. They haven't talked in quite a while. She also sends one of her favorite girlfriends a text and arranges a lunch date for two weeks down the road.

For lunch, she goes to her favorite place outside to eat what she brought. Sometimes, she still goes out to eat with her co-workers, and these days, she almost always chooses a salad with protein in it instead of a burger and fries. She tries to get in as many veggies as she can.

An hour or two after lunch, she drinks another Ningxia Red (her superfood antioxidant) and a Nitro (B vitamins) supplement and gets a nice uplift for the afternoon. She's been sipping on her 32-ounce water bottle all day long and has almost finished her second one by 5 p.m. when she leaves.

She gets home, throws on her comfy clothes, sits on her yoga mat, and does about 20 minutes of stretching. It feels so good after sitting all day in a chair. She heads to the kitchen, takes out some fish, and puts it in the toaster oven with spices and olive oil on top. While that is cooking, she makes some spiral zucchini sauteed in olive oil with salt and pepper. She might also reheat the cooked, cubed sweet potato she has from doing her meal prep at the beginning of the week.

Fifteen minutes later, she and her husband are eating the healthy dinner she had planned the weekend before. The decisions had already been made. Her husband is also grateful for the healthy meal.

She has decided to dedicate an hour after dinner to her newest idea. She has been delving into pottery over the last couple of years, and she wants to teach pottery classes for other women at the local shop. She needs to decide on her curriculum. She also needs to write out all the tasks and tools necessary. She wonders if someday she might be able to buy the pottery shop. The owner is looking to move away in the next two years to be closer to her family.

Bonnie goes to bed an hour earlier than she used to. She is excited to get in bed early, either with her book or maybe a little TV to end the night. Either way, it's been a great day. She is happy, and her family is happy for her. In fact, her children are inspired. She has read up on how to have great relationships with adult children, and she talks to them much more now. They have even started up a weekly Sunday family board game night.

She takes her water bottle to bed and uses it to take her nighttime supplements from one of the baggies stored in her nightstand. She looks forward to her weightlifting tomorrow, knowing how important it is to really focus on building muscle. Good thing it is never too late for this! Excited about her future, she falls asleep easily because she has treated her body and mind well today.

I think we all would prefer to be more like the second Bonnie than the first Bonnie. It's definitely achievable. If Joan MacDonald didn't start lifting weights and getting healthy until she was 70 and still completely transformed her life, we all have the potential for great health at any age!

Let's look again at the rules we need to adhere to as we launch into these sixty days.

Reminder: The Sixty-Day Dare Rules

BodyWork: Pick One for All 60 Days

EAT – On a basic level, you should simply eat a clean diet. That means no alcohol, no desserts, candy, etc. You could add the elimination of processed foods, too, if you want. You may want to do an elimination diet of no wheat or no dairy and see how your body reacts. You may want to add certain things to your diet, like vegetables, fruits, or a certain amount of protein each day. You can also go on a specific diet that you like — but make sure it's a healthy one and not a fad diet.

DRINK – At the minimum, drink ½ your body weight in ounces of water. You will have to keep that water bottle with you at all times.

MOVE – Exercise at least 45 minutes a day. (If you need to start with less, that's fine — but decide on the number of minutes per day that you will do.) Our biggest focus should be on lifting weights, building that muscle, and walking.

SLEEP – Get seven to nine hours of sleep a night. This means you'll need to plan to get to bed on time, consistently, each night.

BREATHE – Do at least 10 minutes of focused deep breathing a day.

BrainWork: Pick One for All 60 Days

WRITE – Take at least 10 minutes a day to write.

READ – Read at least 10 pages in your book a day (or listen to one podcast or decide on the equivalent length of time for an audiobook – finish the book or podcast).

CLEAR – Devote at least 15 minutes a day to decluttering and/or detoxing your home.

MEDITATE – Pray, meditate, or do affirmations for at least 10 minutes a day.

CREATE – Devote at least 30 minutes a day to your creative endeavor.

WorldWork: Pick DREAM or Rotate Among Any or All Five

DREAM – Write the answer to one DREAM question per day in a journal. (For the 60 Dream questions, see Appendix B.)

ENGAGE – Have a positive, intentional connection with family, friends, or other relationships. This means a conversation back and forth, on the phone, in person, or on video chat, not just via text.

GATHER – Go to something spiritual, such as a gathering, event, small group, intimate get-together, book club, church, one-on-one meeting, etc.

HELP – Volunteer to help anyone with anything and enjoy yourself.

ACT – Spend an hour or more on your mission, vision, or purpose if you know what it is, or try something new on for size.

Since you can choose to rotate among these, **decide during Sunday Planning (see this process below) what you will do each day** for the week.

Tools for Success

Alrighty, my friend. How are you? I want to give you a big hug! This is going to be great! Are you good with everything? Have you set yourself up for success? Is this going to completely stress you out, or have you balanced it all out? Remember, this is the beginning of a new way of doing things, or maybe it's just tweaking things to make them a little better. Either way, you are heading in the right direction. Up!

To help you succeed, here are some general tools that I think everyone needs.

A Written Daily Plan

To do your Sixty-Day Dare successfully, you will need a written plan in some form. You may have a habit tracker app on your phone that works for you, or you may need a written planner that you can look at daily. Life typically just gets too hectic not to have a written plan for you to interact with each day. You will want to check things off to make sure you did what you said you would do. Checking things off is extremely satisfying! You will need to either keep it with you or have it in a place you see daily. (Get the *Reignite! Sixty-Day Dare Planner* from my website at AllisonMcCuneDavis.com.)

Sunday Planning Each Week

I've always liked planning my week on Sunday afternoon or evening. However, I got this more specific idea from one of my coaches, Edie Wadsworth, and I love it.

Part 1: Brain Download of To-Dos

On **Sunday**, sit down and do a **brain download on paper** of all the things you need to do for the coming week, including your Sixty-Day Dare activities, of course. Make that list.

If there's anything on the list that you don't have to do yourself, circle it and put the name of the person to whom you will **delegate** it (spouse, child, someone else).

Is it a **project** that entails a number of different tasks? If so, write that down in a different "project area" and list all the tasks. Delegate some if you can. Add some to your brain download list for this week. Maybe add some to next week.

Is there anything that would be okay to put on next Sunday's planning page instead of this week's? You are not procrastinating here; it would simply be better the next week.

Part 2: Meal Planning

Plan your dinners for the week, and write them on a list. Make it simple. Broiled fish, broccoli, salad. That simple. Think about what you have in the fridge or what you'll need to buy. Maybe you'll go out one night, or maybe you'll have leftovers.

Now your decisions have been made. Next, you will plug each and every item in on the various days of the week.

Part 3: Time Planning

Plan your appointments first. These are things with a **time attached** to them, like a dentist or hair appointment or a job. You will need to make sure you stop making appointments during the important self-care time that you have prioritized. For instance, I never make appointments in the morning for that reason. Only in the afternoons.

Plan your important free time next. Plug into your daily plans for the week when you will work out, when you will plan your week, when you will meal prep, and when you will do your morning and evening routines. When will you do your Sixty-Day Dare items? This is about designing the life you love, not just letting it happen by accident.

Next, **batch like things together.** Errands on the same day. Emails and other computer actions at the same time. Cooking multiple meals at the same time.

Now go back to your brain download, and **plug any other items into your daily calendar pages for the**

week. You are making all the decisions now. Not later. Make sure to leave buffer room and travel time between tasks.

This is the key:

As one of Edie's coaches advised: The Sunday Planning version of you is in charge all week. The decisions have been made. The Wednesday version of you (tired and cranky) doesn't get to change the plan. Your Wednesday self is like a terrorist, and **we don't negotiate with terrorists**. Your Sunday version is smart and knows what she is doing. Obey her.

This is about keeping your word to yourself. Practice this. Your confidence and self-image will improve as you do it. Eventually, you will stop feeling behind all the time and start feeling like you have room in your life and that things are improving.

> *This is about keeping your word to yourself.*

Design Your Ideal Week

The last planning tool that has helped me is to design your ideal week using blocks of time (see Figure 13.1). Blocks of time give you wiggle room and help you set the boundaries necessary to live the life you want to live. As life changes, this "ideal week" will change. Life is never perfect, but seeing your goal for the ideal week regularly will, little by little, help you get there. Here is an example of mine. Draw up your own.

My Ideal Week

	MONDAY	TUESDAY	WEDNESDAY	THURSDAY	FRIDAY	SATURDAY	SUNDAY
6 AM	Sleep Goal 8-9 Hours						
7 AM	Coffee, Walk, Plan, Design, Podcasts, Read, Oils, Supps, Meditate, Deep Breathing, Get in the Sun						
8 AM							
9 AM						Coffee with Matt	
10 AM	Focused Work						
11 AM	Pilates	Weights	Pilates	Weights	Pilates		Church
12 PM							
1 PM	Focused Work & Appointments					Relax	Relax
2 PM						Fun	
3 PM	Carpool & Kids					Self Care	Lunch or Dinner with Family
4 PM							
5 PM							
6 PM	Cook & Eat	Date with Matt	Cook & Eat	Social	Cook & Eat		Plan Week
7 PM	Walk & Relax with Matt				Walk & Relax with Matt		
8 PM	Bedtime Routine						
9 PM							

Figure 13.1 Ideal Week Example

Remember to Set up Your Environments

You've heard me talk about this multiple times, so I won't go into detail again. Just do everything you can to make your environment trigger the behavior you are looking for.

People Can Help

My biggest dream is for groups of people to read this book and engage in the Sixty-Day Dare together, encouraging and helping each other along the way. So why not ask a few people if they would like to do this with you? It will definitely help!

Remember that phrase: You are the five people you hang out with the most. If, when you think about who those five people are currently, it is not a good thought, then you may need to cultivate new people in your world. The Sixty-Day Dare would be a good way to do it.

Also, as you are setting up your Dare and thinking about what your weeks will look like, if you need help, ask. It would be a really good idea to let the other people in your home know exactly what you are doing so they can, hopefully, be supportive. Tell them how important it is to you to do this.

Also, look at the list of what you want to accomplish. Is there anything on your list you want to ask someone about? Maybe you know people who have experience, and you could get their advice. We all tend to hesitate to reach out to others when we need something. Muster some courage and do it. You will most likely be pleasantly surprised.

Q & A

What if I get sick?

Of course, it depends on what you're doing in your Dare and how sick you actually are, but you do what you can do.

If you can still do all the things, then go for it. If not, then take a few days off. It's not the end of the world. Building new habits takes time.

Also, when we start doing new things for our health, our body might not be used to it and might feel a little worse before it feels better. Be patient. This is normal. Know that it will get better. The body heals. Allow that to happen.

What if I'm traveling?

This is part of your planning. Think it through. When I was doing 75 Hard, several times I did my 45-minute walk all around the airport waiting for the plane. You can almost always find a way to walk if that is what you are doing.

You will have to do more planning on food consumption, but it is not hard to find healthy food in restaurants or grocery stores. Just make a plan, and make sure you create time in your schedule to carry it out.

If you are working on CLEAR, you can declutter your phone or laptop, and you can research what you will purchase for clean, chemical-free products for your home. You can watch an episode of Home Edit on Netflix and get inspired.

If you are working on CREATE, maybe you read a book or watch some YouTube videos about how to get better at your endeavor while you are away if it's something you cannot travel with.

The rest should be pretty easy to do, whether home or away.

What if I have an unsupportive family?

This can be a tough one, but I still believe you can do it.

First, though, have a heart-to-heart talk with your family members and let them know how important this is to you. When you come from a humble, sincere place, it is hard to combat.

Also, it will be even more important for you to find outside support. Friends, extended family, a church, a group, etc. Make the effort to reach out and find others. Honestly, once your family sees you improving yourself, as long as you aren't badgering them to join you, it is usually impressive and motivating to them.

Finalize Your Sixty-Day Plan

Write out your plan. Make several copies. Post it in all of the places you regularly see. Tape it to the bottom of your computer screen. On the fridge. On your makeup mirror. Create it as a wallpaper on your phone.

You are amazing, and I'm so proud of you already!

CHAPTER 14

The Sixty-Day Dare and Beyond

Success is not final; failure is not fatal:
it is the courage to continue that counts.
— UNKNOWN

I love that quote. It really encapsulates how we should think every day. It's another way to say, "Take those baby steps and gather your courage to try something new." Just focus on that.

Remember, this first time is your start. You may decide to do several sets of Sixty-Day Dares, up-leveling each time. I mentioned earlier that habits generally require two to eight months to solidify, depending on various factors. That is why "Sixty Is a Good Start!"

Tiny Things Make a Difference

You never know what little idea will really make something work for you or make it more doable. It's so funny. My husband agrees with me on this. We have both been to sooooo many conferences over the years on business and, for me, on natural health. We've realized that many of the key insights we have taken away from a several-day conference happen when we are at lunch or dinner with other participants, and those people share their tips or tricks that helped them.

See the *Reignite!* toolkit page in the back of the book to get tips beyond what's here in this book. Maybe you'll find something there that sparks another idea on how you can make your Sixty-Day Dare even more of a success.

Give Someone Permission

I have done this for decades. Ask someone close to you to call you out when you speak the words that are not what you really want to speak. Over the years, I've said to various friends, "Hey, if you hear me own a sickness or speak words that are not what I want in my life, call me out on it. I give you permission to do that."

This is so helpful. It is easy to not notice how we speak. We are retraining ourselves now. It will take attention, but I know you can do it!

Then and Now

As I think back to my experience with 75 Hard and how it changed me, I am amazed. I am so much more tuned in to daily exercise and also drinking enough water each day. A few months after 75 Hard, I did two more 30-day challenges associated with it. All of that was about three years ago, and it has had lasting effects. I'm excited to continue my own Sixty-Day Dares to keep up-leveling the key longevity areas of my life. I'm excited for you to do the same for your life.

Do You Need a Community?

You will need to determine what your specific situation lends itself to. You might decide to take this on by yourself. Maybe the accompanying Sixty-Day Dare Planner would benefit you, or maybe you have a system already in mind with a favorite planner, notebook, or app. That's wonderful! Go for it!

You might decide to ask your spouse, significant other, friend, or a group of friends to do this with you. You can discuss amongst yourselves how you will keep track of things or how you will proceed together. You each may have your own system, or you may all decide to use the same system. I recommend you chat often and keep track of how everyone is doing.

In my family, I am definitely the one who wants to discuss all the different health topics. That is probably obvious. (My kids are rolling their eyes right now, for sure!) However, every time I have ever told my husband something like, "Hey, I'm going to start focusing on protein and veggies," or

"Hey, I'm going to start walking every day for 45 minutes," he always, without fail, says, "I'll do it with you."

The point here is not that he is such a great husband (though he is!). The point is that if you said this to the people in your circle, some might want to join you. People are often just looking for someone to lead them to something good, something that will benefit them, something that will improve their life, something that will be easier with two or more.

See if someone would like to do this Sixty-Day Dare with you. I really believe this is a key. So, I urge you to find that person or group of people to join you.

Sixty-Day Dare Group Program

If you can't get anyone to do it with you, or even if you can, you might also like to join our Sixty-Day Dare program, where I will be doing it with you and with others like you. It will be a wonderful way to connect and make new friends too. See the page for the *Reignite!* toolkit at the end of the book on how to join.

60 Days from Now

These sixty days are going to change your life in ways you can't even begin to comprehend right now. They will be transformative and will redefine your outer limits, remold your mindset, and

These sixty days are going to change your life in ways you can't even begin to comprehend right now.

232

revitalize your zest for life. You will be unlocking a new version of yourself.

You will experience days of initial excitement, ups and downs in enthusiasm along the way, and ultimately, a powerful push toward the end. Move through those down moments, remembering that they are normal. These stages will teach you lessons of perseverance, self-discipline, and your ability to readjust and adapt.

You will also learn to push through various obstacles, manage your time better, and prioritize tasks that line up with your core values and ultimate objectives. These skills will help in other areas of your life too. Know that a host of different feelings will occur, and remember, they will pass. Just stay the course. (Maybe post that last sentence on your fridge.)

Just stay the course.

This Is Just the Beginning

You will want to continue your education in the areas of BodyWork, BrainWork, and WorldWork. Those resources are right at your fingertips. See my lists of favorite books and podcasts in the *Reignite!* toolkit.

You will also, hopefully, want to continue doing Sixty-Day Dares, up-leveling your life in the three areas. It's a great way to create new habits in bite-size chunks.

When you've finished this Sixty-Day Dare and those new habits are going well, do another Sixty-Day Dare with all new habits to add on top. I know it sounds crazy right now. Have faith: It won't later!

Once you see what the first one has done for you, you will want to keep going. When you do, I'll be your biggest cheerleader. Let me know how it goes by joining me on social media or sending me an email through the channels listed on my About the Author page. I can't wait to hear your story!

Stay the course, but adjust
Stay yourself, but evolve
Stay humble, but lead
Stay hungry, but be grateful
Stay focused, but explore
Stay awake, but dream
— EDDIE PINERO

Epilogue

Not everyone makes it to sixty. As I was finishing this book, my dear 54-year-old youngest sister, Louisa, passed away. She played a significant and wonderful role in my life and in the world, and I miss her so much. What a reminder of what a privilege it is to live to sixty and beyond. Let's make it count!

Acknowledgements

This book is only possible because of the years of work from the longevity researchers I've talked about. Dan Buettner, Gary Young, ND, Jason Prall, Dr. Kelly Turner, and other researchers and scientists.

Thank you to the many mentors and teachers I have had along the way. Some are my friends, and others are those whose written work has taught me much. I certainly wouldn't be here without you!

These amazing people include Catherine Rott, Carrie McVige, Jennifer Travis, Julie Davis, Alice Reynolds, Dr. Michael Leu, Kelly Wright, Emily Buller, Debra Starkey, Sera Johnson, Judy Masters, Mary Young, Shauna VanBogart, Chalene Johnson, Edie Wadsworth, Dr. William Davis, Weston A. Price, Marcella Von Harting, Ray Higdon, Jesse Itzler, Andy Frisella, Wim Hof, Dr. Mark Hyman, Joan McDonald, James Clear, Dr. Vonda Wright, Dr. Casey Means, Bo Eason, Roy Vaden, and Rob Garibay.

Also, a huge thank you to Nicole Gebhardt at Niche Pressworks for showing me a better way to write this book, and to her wonderful team for helping me get it to the finish line.

Most of all, thank you, reader, for spending your most precious resource, time, to read this book. I pray for your success.

Sixty-Day Dare Planning Sheet

Sixty-Day Dare at a Glance

BODYWORK

Choose 1 for 60 Days

- ☐ **EAT** – My plan is _____
- ☐ **DRINK** _____ oz/day (Rec*: 1/2 bodyweight in oz)
- ☐ **MOVE** _____ min/day (Rec: 45 min)
- ☐ **SLEEP** _____ hrs/night (Rec: 7-9 hrs)
- ☐ **BREATHE** _____ min/day (Rec: 10 min)

BRAINWORK

Choose 1 for 60 Days

- ☐ **WRITE** _____ min/day (Rec: 10 min)
- ☐ **READ** _____ pages/day (Rec: 10 pages)
- ☐ **CLEAR** _____ min/day (Rec: 15 min)
- ☐ **MEDITATE** _____ min/day (Rec: 10 min)
- ☐ **CREATE** _____ min/day (Rec: 30 min)

WORLDWORK

Choose Dream for 60 Days or Rotate Daily Your Choice

- ☐ **DREAM** _____ question(s) per _____
- ☐ **ENGAGE** – interaction w/another _____ per week
- ☐ **GATHER** – attend a spiritual event _____ per week
- ☐ **HELP** – volunteer activity _____ per week
- ☐ **ACT** _____ min/day (Rec: 60 min) _____ days/weeks

*Rec = Recommended

APPENDIX B

The Sixty-Day Dare DREAM Questions

Use these to do the DREAM option of WorldWork in the Sixty-Day Dare. Even if you're not doing the DREAM option, you can also just journal about them as you like for the benefit of discovering more about yourself and your purpose in the world.

1. As you start the process of dreaming about this part of your life, what are the first thoughts that come to mind when I ask you the question, "What are the innermost dreams you may have had your entire life, that still tug at your heart?"

2. What worldly issues break your heart so much that when they come up in conversation, you definitely have something to say?

3. What worldly issues make you angry, and with the right people, you will totally rant on the subject and all of the details?

4. What have you done in your life where you were so engrossed you didn't notice the time passing? It could be anything. Crafting? Woodworking? Mentoring? Making something? Cooking? Working out? Working with animals? Putting on makeup? Renovating homes? Painting? Volunteering? Reading? Writing? The possibilities are endless.

5. How would you describe your identity today? Who are you? What do you do? What do you enjoy?

6. Think way back to your years as a child, from ages one to eighteen. It may be hard, but close your eyes and put yourself there. What did you love or love to do as a child? What about in your teen years? Did you have any ideas of what you might like to be when you grew up? Who or what did you admire at that time?

7. Do you know what your name means? First, middle, and last? Knowing the meaning of your name can help identify your purpose in life. I am amazed at how, sometimes, the meaning of someone's name directly correlates to part of their purpose or their core values. My

favorite book for looking up names is *The Name Book* by Dorothy Astoria. If you find a negative meaning, flip it to the opposite. You can also do an online search. Write down any insights here.

8. It's amazing how we can go back to an experience, a period in our lives, maybe in childhood or early adulthood, and pinpoint something that started it all. It could have been something positive or negative. Do you know what that one thing is for you? Sit down, close your eyes, put on some meditative music, and think back. What are some possibilities? Write them down.

9. We are all here to help others in some way. We are all connected, and we each have experiences we have come through that can help someone else. In many cases, such experiences become our life purpose. Think back to times when you struggled. Those difficult times in your life. What have you overcome? Did you have a difficult childhood? What have you come through to make it to the other side? Make a list here of those things. This is a possible lead to your purpose.

10. Go back to the decade of your twenties. Describe what you were doing and what your dreams and aspirations were at that time. Describe the skills and talents you might have been developing. Were you starting to do what you truly wanted to be doing? Why or why not? What were your dreams at that time?

11. Who do you want to be now? Fit? Athletic? Healthy? A writer? A speaker? An awesome mother or grand-mother, a master gardener, a pilot, a course-creator, a painter, an entrepreneur, a chess champion, a musician? Maybe it's multiple things. Brainstorm all the possibilities. Even the ones you are not sure about, and list them all right here. Be brave. Write every-thing down, even the things you fear or don't think are possible.

12. What activities make you come alive?

13. What kind of people do you like to hang out with? Describe them.

14. If you have a significant other or spouse, what is it about them that made you want to be with them? What attracted you to them in the first place?

15. What did you love most about your parents or a paren-tal figure in your life? Discuss their qualities.

16. What do you look forward to most in your week?

17. List the last few times that you felt extremely happy.

18. List the ten coolest things about you. The list can en-compass anything you have done, seen, or become in your life. They can be small things or big things. Who are you truly? Who are you authentically? So many of us brush off the remarkable things about ourselves as

no big deal. We minimize them because, to us, they are just what we do or what we did. However, to many others, the things we do can appear amazing and so different from what they do.

19. List your five favorite movies of all time. Often, a common theme runs through them. What is that theme? What is similar about these movies? A theme that runs through your life is likely a similar theme that runs through your favorite movies. What might that be, and what might it say about you? Maybe you'd prefer to list your five favorite books and do the same exercise. Choose one or both.

    As an example, I'll show you my list:

    - *Braveheart*
    - *Gladiator*
    - *Gone With the Wind*
    - *The Matrix*
    - *The Woman King*

    The theme I keep coming up with is a reluctance of the main character to do what they end up doing or what they know deep down they should do. I feel that reluctance — the desire to just stay safe in my home, introverting. But no. We can't do that. We must step out and fulfill our true purpose.

20. Core Values, Step 1: I predict you probably have done some self-development through the years. Regardless of how much you have done or whether you have done

exercises like these before or not, things change over time. Our dreams and desires can change. Our life circumstances change. We have revelations about new directions in our lives. Right?

I've done these exercises multiple times, and it seems that each time has helped me narrow down more specifically who I am and what I really want deep inside. Everyone's core values about the most important things are different from everyone else's. Thank God for that! No answer is more right or better than any others. The goal here is to narrow down what your top five core values are.

Here is a list of ideas. Go through this list and start by putting a check mark by all the words that resonate as important to you. Check as many as you want, but we will be engaging in a narrowing-down process, so the fewer you pick, the easier that will be as we move forward. If you have a word that is not on this list, add it and check it. You can also search the internet for more "core value words."

Abundance	Accountability	Authenticity
Achievement	Adaptability	Adventure
Authority	Autonomy	Balance
Beauty	Boldness	Compassion
Challenge	Change	Citizenship
Charisma	Clarity	Committed
Community	Competency	Confidence
Consistent	Contribution	Courageous
Creativity	Credibility	Curiosity
Decisiveness	Delight	Dependability

Determination	Educating	Efficient
Empathy	Encouragement	Enthusiasm
Excellence	Fairness	Faith
Fame	Family	Friendships
Fun	Generosity	Growth
Happiness	Hard Work	Honesty
Honor	Hope	Humor
Humble	Imagination	Independence
Influence	Ingenuity	Innovation
Harmony	Important Work	Inspiring
Integrity	Intimacy	Intuition
Justice	Kindness	Knowledge
Laughter	Leadership	Learning
Love	Loyalty	Management
Nurturing	Openness	Optimism
Organization	Partnership	Passionate
Patience	Peace	Persistence
Planning	Pleasure	Poise
Popularity	Positive	Power
Professionalism	Prosperity	Quality
Recognition	Reliability	Religion
Reputation	Resourceful	Respect
Responsibility	Security	Self-Control
Self-Discipline	Self-Respect	Service
Socializing	Spirituality	Spontaneity
Stability	Status	Success
Support	Sustainability	Teamwork
Tidiness	Transparency	Travel
Trustworthiness	Truth	Wealth
Wellness	Wisdom	

21. Core Values, Step 2. Now, go back and narrow that list down to only ten words. Underline the ten words that are most important to you. I know it's hard to do, but by focusing on it, you can narrow it down.

22. Core Values, Step 3. For the final process, go back one more time and circle the top five words that are most important to you. Great job! Now, you have your top five core values.

    These are very important words for you to keep in the forefront of your mind as often as possible. Use them as you think of the branding for a business you might want to start, for the next project you want to work on, for the next vacation you want to go on, or for the next time you want to teach your children or grandchildren something important about life. Put them on a sticky note, and place it where you will see it.

    Remember the idea of "only do what only you can do" and that time is short. Use these words as your guidepost for how you spend your days.

23. Timeline: Turn a piece of paper so the long side is horizontal. Draw a horizontal line across the page in the middle, so you have space above and below it. This is your life to date. Put a mark on the line for every five to ten years. Then plot the defining moments of your life on this timeline. There will be some positive ones. Put those above the line. The better the moment, the higher above the line it is plotted. There will be some negative and some awful. Plot those below the line. The worse the moment, the lower you plot it. This timeline of the

defining moments of your life will be useful as you continue down the path of realization and actualization. Write down any insights.

24. Find Your "One True Sentence," Step 1. I love this exercise from Bo Eason, a speaking coach. Obviously, this is not a course on speaking to an audience. I think this exercise can simply be instructive in knowing yourself better. Of the defining moments of your life, can you pick one that was the *most* defining? If not, just choose one for this exercise.

   Write, stream of consciousness, what happened. How did you feel? What did you see and smell? Why was it significant? Did it cause you to make a major decision to do something or to not do something ever again? Did you decide to fight, or lead, or do something else significant? How did it change you? How did this experience make you who you are today?

   No judgment, just write.

25. One True Sentence, Step 2: Take your One True Sentence a step further and rewrite this story from another person's point of view talking about you. This person is a parent, sibling, coach, teacher, etc. It's someone who likes you very much and has made a significant impact on your life. Tell the story as if that person is telling it about you.

26. One True Sentence, Step 3: Now, from a 3rd person point of view, to bring greater significance to your story, write it as a fairy tale. You could start with something like "Once upon a time in a land far, far away there was a beautiful young maiden..." or similar.

27. One True Sentence, Step 4: Now, create your One True Sentence from your story. Put your story into just one true sentence. Bo told us this is how Hemingway would start writing when he was stuck. He would just write one true sentence about something, and then he would be off. Write down your One True Sentence.

    When I did this exercise, my one true sentence was this: "After almost killing myself on my solo flight, I vowed to never ignore my intuition again." Turns out "intuition" is one of my core values.

28. What do you naturally do well that others come to you for advice or help with?

29. What are your strongest abilities, talents, and skills today?

30. What is one thing you could do every day even if no one paid you?

31. What do you do for fun?

32. What do you do that is fulfilling to your soul?

33. What thing do you do now, or did you do in the past, and you had no idea how much time passed? You looked up, and you thought thirty minutes had passed when several hours had gone by. This is a key to what you may love. This is "flow." Our zone of genius can have much to do with when we get into "flow."

34. What kinds of causes and people are you drawn to? What things make you angry in the world? What breaks your heart? What gets you on a soapbox with someone who thinks as you do, and you don't have to worry about offending them? What do you get riled up about having or doing? If you aren't sure, do some journaling anyway, then go through another week or so of everyday life and notice when something triggers you. Make notes about it right then.

35. What topics are you most passionate about?

36. If you had a message to the world, what would that be? What do you believe so strongly in? Maybe it was something you said repeatedly to your children as they grew.

37. Brainstorm some ways you could use your abilities to serve others around a topic that is of great interest to you.

38. If you could work with one person on a project, describe that person in detail. Age, gender, lives in what city, family status, education level, personal interests, values, and characteristics in detail.

39. Think of someone who thinks you are awesome and helpful to them. Describe them.

40. Why would you like to work with the person you described above?

41. How could your interests (could be several) serve this kind of person?

42. Make a list of five to ten problems this kind of person has.

43. What are three big challenges you can help them with?

44. What is the one top-of-mind problem you could aim to solve for them?

45. What are their other options for solving this problem?

46. What do they really want? (Peace of mind, security, a purpose, a plan, fun, escape)

47. Now, for fun, let's create something those starting a business are smart to do. Even if you are simply looking for direction, this can help.

    To create a Value Proposition, look at the information you have been brainstorming and put it into one statement. You may hone this statement over time, changing it a bit here and a bit there as you grow and change. Try it here.

    I am a _____ *(my role)* _____ and I help _____ *(my target market)* _____ to do/ understand _____ *(my unique solution)* _____ so that _____ *(the transformation I provide)* _____.

    Here is mine as an example:

I am a *wife, mom, entrepreneur, and author* and I help *women in the second part of life* to *get healthy naturally, understand the purpose of their life, and reignite that passion* so that *they can have peace of mind, joy, and knowledge that they will have a life well-lived*.

48. Create a short, catchy brand slogan or tagline from your sentence above. Here is an example.

    Example: "Helping women over fifty get healthy, find their purpose, reignite their passion, and know they will have a life well-lived."

    What could yours be? Don't worry. You don't have to create a business here, but you sure could. Again, we are solidifying you and your purpose in the world. Try a few different versions.

49. Here is another way to look at why you want to do what you want to do. According to Gazelles, Verne Harnish's business consulting company, there are four types of Core Purpose for any business.

    1. Service to others
    2. Search for knowledge and truth
    3. Pursuit of beauty and excellence
    4. Desire to change the world

    I believe these are also core purpose categories for any person, and though they all can be important, we can probably each fit our purpose mostly into one of these areas.

If you are a researcher and writer, maybe your purpose is #2. If you are a health care giver or volunteer, maybe it is #1. If you are an artist of any sort or a designer, maybe it is #3. If you are pursuing a non-profit organization or an inventor or selling an exciting new product, maybe it is #4. You can certainly feel that you are all four of these or any combination too. Just identifying where you are here is homing in on who you are and what your purpose is.

For your exercise, re-order these four types of core purpose in the order of importance to you in your life. Which goes in spots #1, #2, #3, and #4.

50. Another type of business exercise is a SWOT Analysis in which you identify Strengths, Weaknesses, Opportunities, and Threats. From your heart, answer these questions about your life. What are your top five in each category?

- What are your Strengths?
- What are your Weaknesses?
- What are your current Opportunities?
- What are your Threats? (Not what is necessarily happening now, but what could happen if you aren't vigilant in key areas of your life?)

51. Alignment exercise, Step 1: I love this simple alignment exercise I learned from Shauna VanBogart. Make a list of your current 1) goals and visions, 2) major areas where you spend your time, and 3) major thoughts you have for your life. List everything that is currently taking up space in your mind.

52. Alignment exercise, Step 2: Go back through each entry in your list and place it into one of the three following categories to indicate how you really feel about it, deep down, in your physical body.

   a. Fully Aligned: This item feels expansive, and no matter what, you know you want it, you are up for it, it is good, and you want it to happen!
   b. Semi-Aligned: You're unclear. One day, it feels like the right thing; the next day, it doesn't quite feel that way.
   c. Misaligned: Your body feels restrictive when you think about this one. Maybe it was a good idea at one point, but now, maybe not so much. You feel some resistance in your body when you think about it. You might think, "maybe later, but not now."

53. Alignment exercise, Step 3. Go back to your assessment in the above exercise:

   a. Write about how you can increase your pursuit of the fully aligned areas.
   b. Write about what you should do about the semi-aligned areas to get them into one of the other two categories if possible. Or maybe they just need to stay where they are for now.
   c. Write about how you could change or eliminate those misaligned areas.

54. The Talk to Myself Exercise. This exercise shows how the mind can mess with you but can also make that

beautiful turn to protect and encourage you. Think of something you really want to do but you don't think you can. You will say that thing repeatedly aloud, write it down, and then give your brain's immediate response to your statement each time. Do it over and over until the response begins to have a slight change. Continue until that change gets to where you want it.

As an example, I've used the real moment I decided to write this book.

> *I can't write this book.*
> *You're right, you sure as heck can't.*
> *I can't write this book.*
> *No, you don't have what it takes.*
> *I can't write this book.*
> *Probably not.*
> *I can't write this book.*
> *(Heavy sigh) Probably true.*
> *I can't write this book.*
> *Really?*
> *I can't write this book.*
> *Well, have you ever tried?*
> *I can't write this book.*
> *Heck, maybe you can.*
> *I can't write this book.*
> *Hey, why don't you just try it?*
> *I can't write this book.*
> *I think you can.*
> *I can't write this book.*
> *Heck, yes, you can; a million other people have. If they can, so can you.*

Hmmm. Maybe you're right.
Heck, yes, I'm right!
Ok, I'm gonna give it a try!
Don't just try. Do it!
Ok, I'm gonna do it!

You may have to keep going many more times through that initial statement. I have, for sure! Be persistent and win over your mind.

55. Let's assume you have some idea of things you want to pursue now. Even if you don't, having a good space is important. In fact, it is one of the most important parts. You've heard me say it multiple times: Environment Triggers Behavior.

    Where will the activity take place? What is the state of that place? What needs to happen to make it better or more suitable? Do you need to acquire another location? This could apply to an entire building or house, a block, a city, a country, or maybe just the corner of your favorite room.

    Write about where you would most like to pursue your next project, mission, art, or dream.

56. Write about whether anything needs to happen to improve or change this area so that it is conducive to your success.

57. If you don't have a space, or if it's not perfect, will you allow that to prevent you from pursuing your dreams? Don't get sidetracked by perfection. There is a saying, "Done is better than perfect." How can you just do it anyway?

58. Have you had some revelations as you have gone through these exercises? Even if your new thoughts are still not solidified, write down your best plan for a future you can look forward to. What elements does it include?

People who write down their goals are much more likely to achieve them than people who don't. There is a Bible verse I LOVE about this: "Write the vision and make it plain" (Habakkuk 2:2, NKJV).

Inc.com tells us that 60 percent of people abandon their New Year's resolutions or goals within six months, and 25 percent do so within seven days. If you write your goals down, you are 42 percent more likely to achieve them. So, write it down, for heaven's sake!

59. Your Misogi. Remember that? Mine was 75 Hard several years ago; then it was writing this book. I would love for you to create a Misogi each year. A life-changing event that you will remember for years to come. What could it be? Brainstorm all the ideas you can come up with and choose one for this year or next. Maybe it's the Sixty-Day Dare.

60. You can certainly choose NOT to follow through with any of the plans and ideas you have come up with as you've answered all of these questions, but before you do that, write answers to the following questions.

- What will my life look like if I don't take the steps to improve my health and pursue my dreams?

- What will my kids think?
- What will my significant other think?
- How will I feel when I'm looking back at the end of my life?

I hope those answers inspire you to continue on.

About the Author

Allison McCune Davis is a natural health educator and Traditional
Naturopath. She homeschooled her
children for twenty years, taught
yoga on and off, and pursued entre-
preneurial business in the world of
natural health for the last fourteen
years while raising her family.

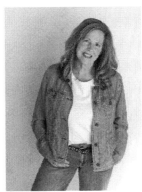

Prior to this, she had a career
as a television producer in Los Angeles. Primary work
included assistant to the creative director for special effects on *Star Trek — The Next Generation*, *Max
Headroom*, and Prince music videos, to name a few. She
served as producer of PBS educational programs and
ABC-TV computer graphics, one of which earned an
LA Emmy Award.

Currently, she is focused on her family and helping
women with holistic health and longevity. She is the wife
of her super-smart lawyer husband, Matthew, and mom
to her five amazing children — Emma, Meg, Henry,
Luke, and Sally — three biological and two adopted
from the beautiful countries of Russia and Ethiopia.

Contact

Instagram: Instagram.com/allison.mccune.davis

Website: AllisonMcCuneDavis.com

Email: Allison@AllisonMcCuneDavis.com

To get *Reignite! The Sixty-Day Dare Planner*, go to my website at AllisonMcCuneDavis.com.

A Small Request

You've probably noticed that I'm on a mission to get everyone healthy and bust the age myths wide open. And I'd like to ask for your help.

If you enjoyed this book and felt it was helpful, could you do me a favor and give me an honest review on Amazon?

Reviews are crucial for authors in getting their books into the right hands. With just a few moments of your time, you could help someone else find this book or decide to buy it — and I would be so grateful for that. And if it helps them, I bet they will be, too.

Thanks in advance for being part of the mission!

—Allison

Download Your
REIGNITE! SIXTY-DAY DARE TOOLKIT

PACKED WITH MORE RESOURCES AND TOOLS TO STAY ON TRACK!

Go to the link below for:

- Tips on dealing with stress and sleep
- Favorite podcasts and books
- Affirmations for various purposes
- Favorite products and sources
- My basic protocol when pushing through a cold or flu
- The Sixty-Day Dare Group Program
- And more!

These will help you with your Sixty-Day Dare and life in general.

HERE'S TO YOUR LONGEVITY!
SPIRIT, SOUL & BODY!
—Allison

AllisonMcCuneDavis.com/Toolkit

Endnotes

Below is the list of references and citations for the book. Science and stats can certainly change over time and may need to be updated. Also, I could easily have made a mistake somewhere in giving credit to the wrong person or not giving credit where it is due. I certainly apologize for that, and if you believe that to be true, please email me at allison@allisonmccunedavis.com so the issue can be fixed.

1   "Jesse Itzler's Big A## Calendar," accessed October 7, 2024, https://jesseitzler.com/pages/calendar.
2   "75 Hard," Andy Frisella, accessed May 8, 2024, https://andyfrisella.com.
3   Caroline Leaf, *Switch on Your Brain: The Key to Peak Happiness, Thinking, and Health* (Grand Rapids, MI: Baker Books, 2013), Page 152.
4   Raindrop Technique® Bodywork, Young Living Essential Oils, accessed October 8, 2024, https://www.youngliving.com/us/en/learn/raindrop-technique.

5   Weston A. Price, DDS, *Nutrition and Physical Degeneration* (Lemon Grove, California: Price Pottenger Nutrition, 2009).

6   Jordan S. Rubin, *The Maker's Diet: The 40-Day Health Experience That Will Change Your Life Forever* (Lake Mary, FL: Siloam, 1982).

7   William Davis, MD, *Wheat Belly: Lose the Wheat, Lose the Weight, and Find Your Path Back to Health* (New York: Rodale, 2011).

8   Mary Young, *Seed to Seal: D. Gary Young* (Lehi, UT: Mary Young, 2015).

9   Young ND, Gary. "Ningxia Wolfberry: The Ultimate Superfood." *Essential Science Publishing*, 2006. Page v.

10 Dan Buettner, *The Blue Zones* (Washington, D.C.: National Geographic, 2012.

11 Buettner, pages 267-295.

12 "Grandma Moses (Anna Mary Robertson Moses)," National Museum of Women in the Arts, accessed October 10, 2024, https://nmwa.org/art/artists/grandma-moses-anna-mary-robertson-moses/#:~:text=At%20 78%2C%20when%20arthritis%20rendered,fireboard%20 for%20her%20first%20paintings.

13 Rachel Gillett and Richard Feloni, "19 Extremely Successful People Who Changed Careers after Turning 30," *Inc.*, November 29, 2017, https:// www.inc.com/business-insider/people-who-found-success-and-changed-careers-after-30-years-old. html#:~:text=Julia%20Child%20worked%20in%20 advertising,a%20celebrity%20chef%20in%201961.

14 Historic Missourians, "Laura Ingalls Wilder," accessed October 12, 2024, https://historicmissourians.shsmo.

org/wilder-laura-ingalls/#:~:text=In%201932%2C%20
at%20the%20age,published%20between%201933%20
and%201943.

15 Bill Murphy, Jr., "14 Inspiring People Who Found
Crazy Success Later in Life," Inc., March 24, 2015,
https://www.inc.com/bill-murphy-jr/14-inspiring-peo-
ple-who-found-crazy-success-later-in-life.html.

16 Noelle Carter, "Roy Choi's mom, 'Mommy Choi,'
Teaches Us How to Make Spicy Korean Rice Cakes,"
February 15, 2018, https://www.latimes.com/food/
dailydish/la-fo-co-roy-choi-mom-cooking-recipe-
20180217-story.html.

17 Abbey Bender, "At 85 and 83, Lily Tomlin and Jane
Fonda Have Been Pals 45 Years — 3 Things Keep
Their Friendship Strong," Yahoo!Life, January 31,
2023, https://www.yahoo.com/lifestyle/85-83-lily-tom-
lin-jane-141615006.html.

18 Abby Carney, "It's Official! 92-Year-Old's Marathon
World Record Finally Approved," Runners World,
August 3, 2023, https://www.runnersworld.com/news/
a44727305/92-year-old-marathon-world-record/.

19 The Foundation for a Better Life, "Nola Ochs Went
Back to College at 95. At 100, She Had Earned
Her Bachelor's and Master's Degrees," The Denver
Gazette, October 10, 2023, https://gazette.com/life/
nola-ochs-went-back-to-college-at-95-at-100-she-
had-earned-her-bachelor/article_df04a732-63b2-11ee-
85c5-0f65ede7d868.html.

20 "Rooting Around: How a Nation Found Its
Way Back to Breastfeeding," La Leche League
International, October 25, 2024, https://llli.org/news/

rooting-around-how-a-nation-found-its-way-back-to-breastfeeding/.

21 On protecting consumers from toxics in cosmetics, U.S. lags at least 80 countries," EWG, October 22, 2024, https://www.ewg.org/news-insights/news/2021/08/protecting-consumers-toxics-cosmetics-us-lags-least-80-countries.

22 Casey Means, MD, *Good Energy: The Surprising Connection Between Metabolism and Limitless Health* (New York: Penguin Random House, January 2024).

23 Frank W. Stahnisch and Marja Verhoef, "The Flexner Report of 1910 and Its Impact on Complementary and Alternative Medicine and Psychiatry in North America in the 20th Century," *Evidence-based Complementary and Alternative Medicine (eCAM)* (2012) 647896, doi:10.1155/2012/647896.

24 Casey Means, MD, *Good Energy: The Surprising Connection Between Metabolism and Limitless Health* (NYC, NY: Penguin Random House, January 2024), p. 63.

25 Harvard University, "Doctors Need More Nutrition Education," T.H. Chan School of Public Health, accessed October 12, 2024, https://www.hsph.harvard.edu/news/hsph-in-the-news/doctors-nutrition-education/#:~:text="Today%2C%20most%20medical%20schools%20in,obscene%2C"%20Eisenberg%20told%20NewsHour.

26 Robin Feldman, "The Problem with Direct-to-Consumer Pharmaceutical Advertising," *The Washington Post,* March 2, 2023, https://www.washingtonpost.com/made-by-history/2023/03/02/drug-advertising-consumers/#.

27 Casey Means, MD, "American Health Is Getting Destroyed (and It Is Simple to Improve)," Newsletter 25, Casey Means MD (blog), August 26, 2024, https://www.caseymeans.com/learn/newsletter-25.

28 John Abramson, *Sickening: How Big Pharma Broke American Health Care and How We Can Repair It,* (New York: HarperCollins/Mariner Books, 2022).

29 Leah Collins, "Job Unhappiness Is at a Staggering All-Time High, According to Gallup," CNBC, August 12, 2022, https://www.cnbc.com/2022/08/12/job-unhappiness-is-at-a-staggering-all-time-high-according-to-gallup.html.

30 Eric S. Kim, Koichiro Shiba, Julia K. Boehm, Laura D. Kubzansky, "Sense of Purpose in Life and Five Health Behaviors in Older Adults," Preventive Medicine, 139 (2020):106172, https://doi.org/10.1016/j.ypmed.2020.106172.

31 Dan Buettner and Sam Skemp. "Blue Zones: Lessons From the World's Longest Lived." *American Journal of Lifestyle Medicine,* 10, no. 5 (July 7, 2016): 318-321, doi:10.1177/1559827616637066.

32 Liji Thomas, MD, "Unlocking the Secrets of Blue Zones: A Blueprint for Longevity and Health," News Medical Life Sciences, accessed October 12, 2024, https://www.news-medical.net/health/Unlocking-the-Secrets-of-Blue-Zones-A-Blueprint-for-Longevity-and-Health.aspx#:~:text=Blue%20Zones%20worldwide,-Buettner%20described%20five&text=Ikaria%2C%20a%20small%20Greek%20island,%2C%20and%20live%20stress%2Dfree.

33 A.M. Herskind, M. McGue, N.V. Holm, T.I. Sørensen, B. Harvald, and J.W. Vaupel, "The Heritability of

Human Longevity: a Population-based Study of 2872 Danish Twin Pairs Born 1870-1900," *Human Genetics* 97, no. 3 (1996): 319–23. doi:10.1007/BF02185763.

34 University of Alberta, "Your DNA Is Not Your Destiny – or a Good Predictor of Your Health," *ScienceDaily,* December 19, 2019, www.sciencedaily.com/releases/2019/12/191219142739.htm.

35 Buettner, pages 267-295.

36 "Aiming for Longevity," Harvard Health Publishing, October 25, 2004, https://www.health.harvard.edu/staying-healthy/aiming-for-longevity#:~:text=%22Just%20keep%20going%20and%20going,that%20lead%20to%20better%20health.%22.

37 The Human Longevity Project, *The Secret to Radiant Health Beyond 100,* accessed October 12, 2024, https://humanlongevityfilm.com.

38 Kelly Turner, *Radical Remission: Surviving Cancer Against All Odds* (New York: HarperCollins, 2014), p. 6. A radical remission occurs whenever 1 - A person's cancer goes away without using any conventional medicine; or 2 - a cancer patient tries conventional medicine, but the cancer does not go into remission, so he or she switches to alternative methods of healing, which lead to a remission; or 3 - a cancer patient uses conventional medicine and alternative healing methods at the same time in order to outlive a statistically dire prognosis (i.e., any cancer with a less than 25 percent chance of five-year survival.) Turner traveled to ten countries, from the U.S. to China to Zimbabwe, interviewing alternative medicine healers. She also interviewed over 100 people with cases of radical

remission and analyzed over 1000 written cases. And I'm sure there are others. It's all about our lifestyles.

39 Trinity School Of Natural Health, author's personal notes.

40 Nazik Elgaddal, Ellen Kramarow, and Cynthia Reuben, "Physical Activity Among Adults Aged 18 and Over: United States, 2020," National Center for Health Statistics, August 30, 2022, https://www.cdc.gov/nchs/products/databriefs/db443.htm.

41 Haylie Pomroy, *The Fast Metabolism Diet* (Chatsworth, CA: Harmony 2013).

42 Charles Sanford Porter, MD, *Milk Diet as a Remedy for Chronic Disease* (Long Beach, CA: Press Printing Company, 1911).

43 Bernarr Macfadden, *The Miracle of Milk: How to Use the Milk Diet Scientifically at Home* (Austin, TX: Acres U.S.A, 2011).

44 Gary Young, MD, *Ningxia Wolfberry: The Ultimate Superfood,* 2nd Ed., (Orem, UT: Essential Science, 2006) p. v.

45 Trinity School of Natural Health, author's notes.

46 "The association between daily step count and all-cause and cardiovascular mortality: a meta-analysis," *NIH National Library of Medicine,* October 21, 2024, https://pubmed.ncbi.nlm.nih.gov/37555441/.

47 Robby Berman, "Is Exercise More Effective than Medication for Depression and Anxiety?" *Medical News Today,* March 3, 2023, https://www.medicalnewstoday.com/articles/is-exercise-more-effective-than-medication-for-depression-and-anxiety.

48 Chalene Johnson, Smart Success Conference, Los Angeles, 2016.

49 Mark Hyman, MD, "Why Sleep Is More Important Than Diet — Optimize it Today!" Podcast Episode 487, January 28, 2022, https://drhyman.com/blog/2022/01/28/podcast-ep487/.

50 Wim Hof, *The Wim Hof Method: Activate Your Full Human Potential*, (Louisville, CO: Sounds True, Inc., 2020).

51 Gary Brecka, "Breathwork/Ultimate Human Short," *The Ultimate Human* (podcast), October 26, 2023, https://www.youtube.com/watch?v=gLHemX0IE3I.

52 Gary Brecka, https://www.youtube.com/watch?v=C-KRpRpeyVo.

53 James Nestor, *Breath: The New Science of a Lost Art*, (New York: Riverhead Books, 2020).

54 *The Joe Rogan Experience*, "#1506 – James Nestor," July 2020, https://open.spotify.com/episode/58Drs6tKeuq82hMTbcDC0G.

55 James Nestor, *Breath*, p. 84.

56 This one is my favorite. Get the Wim Hof app for more detailed instructions. https://podcasts.apple.com/us/podcast/the-ultimate-human-with-gary-brecka/id1709740887?i=1000632676156.

57 Molly Murray, "Guest Blog: A Major Health Crisis: The Alarming Rise of Autoimmune Disease," National Health Council, March 28, 2024, https://nationalhealthcouncil.org/blog/a-major-health-crisis-the-alarming-rise-of-auto-immune-disease/?utm_source=caseys-means.beehiiv.com&utm_medium=newsletter&utm_campaign=american-health-is-getting-destroyed-and-it-is-simple-to-improve&_bhlid=a4fa07255bf3

88e316a7d0c98610383b3566db83#:~:text=Data%20
indicates%20that%20autoimmune%20diseases,of%20
3%2D12%25%20annually.

58 James Clear, *Atomic Habits* (NYC, NY: Avery, 2018) page 54.

59 Dodie Osteen, *Healed of Cancer* (Houston, TX: Lakewood Church Publications, 1986).

60 Masaru Emoto, *The Hidden Messages in Water* (Hillsboro, OR: Beyond Words Publishing, Inc. 2001).

61 Turner, *Radical Remission* pp. 252–254.

62 G.A. Tooley, S.M. Armstrong, T.R. Norman, and A. Sali, "Acute Increases in Night-time Plasma Melatonin Levels Following a Period of Meditation," *Biological Psychology* 53, no. 1 (2000): 69-78, doi:10.1016/ s0301-0511(00)00035-1.

63 Turner, *Radical Remission* pp. 252–254, citing Britta K. Hölzel, James Carmody, Mark Vangel, Christina Congleton, Sita M. Yerramsetti, Tim Gard, and Sara W. Lazar, "Mindfulness Practice Leads to Increases in Regional Brain Gray Matter Density," *Psychiatry Research* 191, no. 1 (2011): 36–43, doi:10.1016/j. pscychresns.2010.08.006.

64 "Why Does Time Seem to Speed Up with Age?" *Scientific American,* October 23, 2024, https://www.scientificamerican.com/article/ why-does-time-seem-to-speed-up-with-age/.

65 Julia Cameron, *The Artist's Way: 30th Anniversary Edition* (NYC, NY: TarcherPerigee, 2016).

66 Ian Morgan Cron and Suzanne Stabile, *The Road Back to You: An Enneagram to Self-Discovery* (Downers Grove, IL: InterVarsity Press, 2016).

67 Ian Morgan Cron, *Typology*, https://www.typology-podcast.com.

68 Marie Kondo, *The Life-Changing Magic of Tidying Up* (New York: Ten Speed Press, 2014).

69 *Get Organized with the Home Edit*, Netflix, Released 2020, https://www.netflix.com/search?q=home%20 edit&jbv=81094723.

70 Clea Shearer and Joanna Teplin, *The Home Edit: A Guide to Organizing and Realizing Your House Goals* (New York: Clarkson Potter, 2019).

71 Christopher N Cascio, Matthew Brook O'Donnell, Francis J. Tinney, Matthew D. Lieberman, Shelley E. Taylor, Victor J. Strecher, and Emily B. Falk, "Self-Affirmation Activates Brain Systems Associated with Self-related Processing and Reward and Is Reinforced by Future Orientation," *Social Cognitive and Affective Neuroscience* 11, no. 4 (2016): 621–9, doi:10.1093/scan/nsv136.

72 Girija Kaimal, Kendra Ray, and Juan Muniz, "Reduction of Cortisol Levels and Participants' Responses Following Art Making," *Art Therapy: Journal of the American Art Therapy Association* 33 no. 2 (2016): 74–80, doi:10.1080/07421656.2016.1166832.

73 Dr. Henry Cloud and Dr. John Townsend, *Boundaries: When to Say Yes, How to Say No to Take Control of Your Life* (Updated and Expanded Edition) (Grand Rapids, MI: Zondervan, 2017).

74 Saul McLeod, "Pavlov's Dogs Experiment and Pavlovian Conditioning Response," *Simply Psychology*, February 2, 2024, https://www.simplypsychology.org/pavlov.html.

75 Germaine Copeland, *Prayers That Avail Much: Three Bestselling Works Complete in One Volume, 25th Anniversary Edition* (Tulsa, OK: Harrison House Inc.)

76 Carolyn Mein, *Releasing Emotional Patterns with Essential Oils* (Santa Fe, CA: Vision Ware Press, 2020).

77 *The Home Edit,* Netflix.

78 Sheehan D. Fisher, "5 Benefits of Healthy Relationships," HealthBeat, September 2021, https://www.nm.org/healthbeat/healthy-tips/5-benefits-of-healthy-relationships.

79 Gay Hendricks, *The Big Leap: Conquer Your Hidden Fear and Take Life to the Next Level* (New York: HarperOne, 2010) page 34.

80 Macien Stanley, "3 Crucial Discoveries about Purpose in Life," *Psychology Today,* September 1, 2021, https://www.psychologytoday.com/us/blog/making-sense-chaos/202109/3-crucial-discoveries-about-purpose-in-life.

81 James Clear, *Atomic Habits: An Easy and Proven Way to Build Good Habits and Break Bad Ones* (New York: Avery, 2018).

82 Brian Bosché and Gabrielle Bosché, *The Purpose Factor: Extreme Clarity for Why You're Here and What to Do About It* (New York: Post Hill Press, 2020) page 123.

83 Elizabeth Gilbert, *Big Magic: Creative Living Beyond Fear* (New York: Riverhead Books, 2016) Page 35-36.

84 Javier, Yanguas, Sacramento Pinazo-Henandis, and Francisco José Tarazona-Santabalbina, "The Complexity of Loneliness," *Acta Biomedica Atenei Parmensis* 89 no. 2 (2018): 302–14, doi.org/10.23750/abm.v89i2.7404.

85 Dan Buettner, *The Blue Zones: 9 Lessons for Living Longer from the People Who've Lived the Longest* (Washington, DC: National Geographic Partners LLC, 2008), pp. 287–288.

86 Pew Research Center, "Spirituality Among Americans," December 7, 2023, https://www.pewresearch.org/religion/2023/12/07/spirituality-among-americans/.

87 James Clear, *Atomic Habits.*

88 James Clear, *Atomic Habits* Page 84.

89 Caroline Leaf, *Switch on Your Brain: The Key to Peak Happiness, Thinking, and Health* (Grand Rapids, MI: Baker Books, 2013) Page 152.